1991

America's Welfare State

THE AMERICAN MOMENT
Stanley I. Kutler, Series Editor

★ ★ ★

America's Welfare State
From Roosevelt to Reagan

Edward D. Berkowitz

The Johns Hopkins University Press
Baltimore and London

The Johns Hopkins University Press
701 West 40th Street
Baltimore, Maryland 21211
The Johns Hopkins Press Ltd., London

The paper used in this book meets the minimum requirements
of American National Standards for Information Sciences—
Permanence of Paper for Printed Library Materials,
ANSI Z39.48-1984.

Library of Congress Cataloging-in-Publication Data

Berkowitz, Edward D.
    America's welfare state: from Roosevelt to Reagan / Edward D.
Berkowitz.
        p.   cm.—(The American moment)
    Includes bibliographical references and index.
    ISBN 0-8018-4127-5.—ISBN 0-8018-4128-3 (pbk.)
    1. Social security—United States. 2. Public welfare—United
States. 3. Medical care—United States. I. Title. II. Series.
HD7125.B38   1991
361.973—dc20   90-46424   CIP

For My Parents

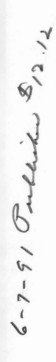

Contents

Series Editor's Foreword

The notions of welfare and a welfare state have aroused passionate conflicts in American life for much of the twentieth century. The Social Security Act of 1935, for example, evoked bitter controversy, perhaps reflected by the Supreme Court's narrowly sustaining the constitutionality of the law two years later. "Constitutionality," of course, was merely a guise for deep-seated policy preferences. Opponents denounced the idea as communistic and subversive of hallowed American traditions of "individualism." Nevertheless, Social Security eventually gained widespread support and by the 1950s moved beyond the pale of political criticism. Indeed, the program has become a fixture, virtually sacrosanct, and political leaders have vied with one another to expand it in response to constituent pressures, not always with beneficial results.

Social Security, as originally conceived, involved citizens, their employers, and government in a joint effort to provide some guaranteed income in people's latter years. Stimulated in part by the Great Depression, advocates of Social Security also saw it as a means for maintaining income and spending for the benefit of the whole society—and at no added governmental cost. Its compulsory feature made it, for many, a welcome alternative to the idea of public dole. Social insurance constitutes the bulk of the welfare state, yet "welfare" resonates as perhaps the most dissonant chord in American public policy. Welfare is commonly distinguished from old-age, survivors, hospital, and disability insurance as a form of governmental handout to the poor, who are believed to be poor because they are lazy, immoral, or both. While such governmental assistance, essentially in the form of Aid to Dependent Children, constitutes a relatively small part of welfare expenditures, it nevertheless receives a disproportionate share of criticism.

Edward Berkowitz offers a masterful understanding of the policies, processes, bureaucracies, and beneficiaries of the welfare state. He has considered the context, impact, and circumstances of such policies as realities, rather than as abstractions. In an even-handed manner, he celebrates the successes of welfare programs and examines their shortcomings. No doubt, Social Security has provided the elderly a "safety net" that was unavailable more than a half-century ago. At the same time, single-parent families and illegitimate births have increased, in some measure because of the accessibility of welfare aid. In other respects, the welfare system has failed for what it has not done, particularly for the lack of a universal and equitable health insurance plan. For Berkowitz, the welfare state is not a palliative to insure social control over a potentially dangerous segment of the population, as some leftist critics have contended, nor has he followed the charges from the right that view the welfare system as a privileged sanctuary for a self-serving bureaucracy and a self-defeating scheme designed to discourage incentive and improvement. Instead, he offers an important historical dimension and a reasoned critique of national welfare programs. With that foundation, we can better consider and improve a system that is a social necessity, yet need not be a social disaster.

Stanley I. Kutler
The University of Wisconsin
Madison, Wisconsin

Preface

Controversial yet little understood, the American welfare state commands little attention from today's students, who view it as a confusing, highly technical, and dry subject that cannot compete with the exploits, often heroic, of the blacks and women who have emerged as major figures in history classrooms over the course of the last twenty years. In the process, various forms of minority studies have somehow subsumed the welfare state as a subject of inquiry. Neither race, nor gender, nor class provides the best frame of reference for understanding the welfare state. I believe the welfare state should be viewed both more broadly, as something that affects all of American society, and more narrowly, as a product of a constricted policy process that limits popular input. In short, I think the welfare state belongs back in the historical mainstream, and this book tries to put it there.

In this historical overview, I trace a general pattern, from conflict in the 1930s and 1940s, to consensus in the 1950s and 1960s, and back to conflict and controversy in the 1970s and 1980s. Contrary to the expectations of today's students, an era once existed in which social welfare programs formed part of a more general consensus that governed American life. Particularly in the years between 1950 and 1965, Americans accepted the key elements of the welfare state. They regarded the Social Security program as a pragmatic approach to the problems of old-age and disability; they did not complain about the lack of comprehensive, governmentally funded national health insurance; and they applauded the creation of a distinctively American approach to health care. They even grudgingly tolerated welfare programs, even though the consensus on this matter began to fray long before criticism of Social Security and American health care became commonplace.

This book contains three major sections, each of which delineates the differences between expectations and outcome that have led to crises in America's welfare state. The first, and longest, section explains the Social Security Act, why Social Security became popular and then almost went bankrupt, and why the policy process appears unable to assure the program's long-term solvency. The second section details the origins of what I call the rehabilitation approach to welfare and the persistence of this approach despite its inability to alleviate what people commonly call the welfare mess. The third section deals with health care and health care cost inflation and shows why, even though we spend twice as much per capita on health care as do the Japanese, so many people do not have health insurance. A final chapter draws conclusions from the three case studies in an effort to come to grips with the crisis of the modern American welfare state.

For most readers, I suspect that words like *welfare, social insurance,* and *welfare state* mean little. Although history represents a sympathetic act of the imagination, even the most astute readers need a brief orientation before they can make the necessary leaps.

It does not help that no one has a good definition of the welfare state. Relying on statistics, one approach posits that when a certain amount of a nation's income—say 8 or 10 percent—gets spent by the government to aid the needy, then a welfare state exists. By this standard, we became a welfare state sometime during the 1950s, when our social welfare expenditures, broadly defined to include such items as Social Security, welfare, health, and education programs, went from 8.2 percent of our gross national product (GNP) (1950) to 10.3 percent (1960). Today we are, by the terms of this definition, deeply entrenched as a welfare state, since we spend about 20 percent of our GNP on social welfare.

Daniel Levine, author of a perceptive study that compares welfare states in various countries, provides another broad-based, if vague, definition of a welfare state. He calls it a "complex, interrelated system of subsidies, tax laws, protective legislation, and income maintenance." As a modern slogan, according to sociologists Edwin Amenta and Theda Skocpol, the term originated during the Second World War in Britain, when it was held up as "an ideal worth fighting for."

I define the term more simply than do Levine, Amenta, or Skocpol. In a welfare state, the government supplies a modicum of security to its citizens, rather than forcing them to rely exclusively on what they earn from working or investing or inheriting.

Welfare represents another confusing concept. At a gut level, most people understand *welfare* to mean a form of government handout. The term evokes an instant shock of recognition and produces an almost visceral reaction. When we think of welfare, we envision a black woman, who lives in a sinister section of the city, miles from the suburbs in which many of us grew up, taking care of her illegitimate children and cashing government checks. When we contemplate welfare, we think of a world like the one portrayed by Spike Lee in the 1989 movie *Do the Right Thing*. Mookie, the movie's hero, delivers pizza in a Brooklyn ghetto. He at least has a job. Most of his friends wander the streets aimlessly, outraging their parents and older relations. Only the owner of the pizzeria, who lives in a white, middle-class section of Brooklyn, and an Oriental family, who manage to make a respectable living from the grocery store across the street, value work. Mookie, who lacks a good job and a clear sense of the future, already has a child, if not a wife. Articulate and blessed with an ironic sense of humor, he stands apart from the rage that seems to grip the younger characters in the movie and the apathy that characterizes the older ghetto residents, who are content to drink wine on the street corner. But he lives in a community in which welfare has become a way of life, in which only outsiders have learned the art of self-sufficiency.

When we consider welfare, we recollect the 1986 Bill Moyers television documentary "The Vanishing Family: Crisis in Black America," featuring interviews with Newark, New Jersey, residents. Once known as the home of novelist Philip Roth, who specialized in writing about Jewish angst, the city now played host to Timothy, a black hedonist who, although a young man, had already fathered six children. He felt little responsibility toward his progeny. Asked whether he should support his children, Timothy told Moyers, "That's on them. . . . I ain't gonna let no woman stand in the way of my pleasures." The show made it abundantly clear that Timothy's children and their mothers would depend on welfare.

While we watch Spike Lee at the movies and Bill Moyers on television, academic writing on this subject laments the lack of a larger welfare state in America. The typical academic exercise involves complicated explanations for why America developed welfare programs so much more slowly than, say, England or Sweden. People's gut impressions simply do not mesh with the available writing on the subject; many people react by ignoring an already unpleasant and confusing subject.

I think the subject needs to be confronted, preferably not with liberal platitudes or conservative pieties but rather through an unromantic, historical account of how we have created our Social Security, welfare, and health insurance programs.

The current intellectual debate over welfare programs serves as a point of departure. Writing for popular audiences, a number of conservatives have demonstrated that America's welfare programs are costly failures, and many liberals simply concede the point. Liberal economist David Ellwood, a professor at Harvard, begins his book on poverty and the American family by explaining why everyone hates welfare. Historian Michael Katz, considerably to the left of most writers on the subject, agrees that "conservatives got far the better part of the argument in the 1980s."

According to Katz, conservatives owed their success to the way in which they defined the agenda in the 1980s. Conservatives, I would argue, simply pointed out the ways in which welfare programs failed to respond to modern conditions. The programs continued to pay mothers to stay home with their children in an era in which women were expected to work. That condition alone, almost by definition, doomed welfare programs to unpopularity. Few people wanted to shell out money and let others "take it easy." Rather than agreeing with this view, many liberals (Ellwood and Katz are two notable exceptions) fell back on a tortured defense of existing welfare programs; so being a liberal came to imply a defensive view of the past rather than a convincing vision of the future. As sociologists Richard Scotch and Edward Harpham noted, in slightly more academic language, "the defining characteristic for a 1980s liberal was no longer a belief in the future possibilities of a benevolent state; it was rather a commitment to the institutions and policies of the New Deal and the War on Poverty."

In the 1980s, backward-looking liberals could not match the glamour and conviction of action-oriented conservatives. Where liberals favored unionization, welfare, training programs, minimum wages, and health and safety regulations as partial solutions to the problems of the black ghetto, conservatives proposed enterprise zones, in which entrepreneurs could enrich themselves and their communities without government hinderance. The conservative agenda for urban development combined an enticing blend of tearing down the old and replacing it with a new idea that appeared to offer hope for the future. Liberals countered that an absence of regulation did not insure the presence of economic growth. Yet they had little to offer in return except more of the same, and the effective criticisms of old programs undermined the appeal of the status quo.

At base, liberals feared that the conservatives simply wanted to dismantle the American version of the welfare state, without offering *anything* in return. Nothing about enterprise zones offered much hope for the characters in Spike Lee's movie or the residents of Bill Moyers's Newark. In the absence of social welfare programs, life only became worse.

How, one wonders, did we get into this situation, in which we rely on old, often self-defeating programs to solve social problems and the policy process offers us a choice between these programs and, in effect, no programs? History helps to answer this intriguing question, particularly when we step back from the academic concerns that have steered scholarship on the American welfare state down blind alleys. Far from confronting conservative critiques or current policy dilemmas, historical writing on the welfare state, as I have already suggested, remains mired in such questions as why some countries initiated welfare states before others and in such esoteric debates as whether "developmental" or "social democratic" forces best explain the welfare state. Neither question advances our understanding of the American welfare state.

Concentrating on the welfare state in international comparison, one risks forgetting that all nations have attempted to cope with poverty and misfortune since the beginning of time. No logic compels one country to follow the lead of another, nor should one country's progress necessarily be measured in terms of another country's accomplishments. It makes more sense to find out what happened in America than to study what did not happen. One needs to know how America handles the problems of financing health care, not why America lacks national health insurance (even though other welfare states do have national health insurance).

The debate over "developmental" or "social democratic" forces has as much to do with the academic preoccupation over the relevance of Marxist theory to social policy as it does with real historical questions about the American welfare state. Believers in developmental forces portray social welfare programs as the natural results of modernization; social democratic forces emphasize the taking of the welfare state from capitalists by means of labor agitation. Neither view adequately explains the development of American social security, welfare, or health care programs.

Both views recognize that as nations industrialize, productivity increases, but so does insecurity. Workers now depend on a wage, whose continuing presence is far from certain, rather than harvesting their own crops or making their own goods. Since industrialism also brings economic growth, some of society's new-found wealth can be spent on reducing a worker's insecurity. The state forces workers to set something aside now to cope with problems later. It pools the workers' "surplus" resources and, in effect, runs an insurance program. The developmental view emphasizes the welfare state as a natural consequence of industrialization; the social democratic view contemplates the welfare state as a benefit that labor wrests from capital.

Whatever the motivation, the results turn out the same. Countries initiate programs that operate like insurance programs in that they substitute a certain small loss for a possible large one. We call such efforts *social insurance*. I. M. Rubinow, an early writer on the subject, defined the term in 1913 as an "effort of the organized state to come to the assistance of the wage-earner and furnish him something he individually is quite unable to obtain for himself." Modern writers equate the welfare state and social insurance.

Good historians, Daniel Levine sensibly argues, dismiss these sorts of compact generalizations; they always want to know more rather than less. Historians realize that, although welfare states may rely on social insurance, they differ from place to place because of differences in national values, cultures, and experiences. As Levine writes, "the history of each country was not isolated—leaders in each of the countries were aware of what was happening in all of the others— but each perceived their neighbors' actions in accordance with their own preconceptions." Levine's view of history, with which I agree, undermines the notion of the welfare state's inevitability and sinks the developmental school.

Labor agitation, the explanation favored by the social democratic school, simply does not describe the American experience. Organized labor played little or no role in the creation of American social insurance programs, symbolized by the passage of the Social Security Act in 1935. Coming from above, rather than below, our welfare state reflected the influence of a small group of social theorists, whom President Roosevelt brought to Washington, not the agitation of workers or labor unions. Furthermore, no reason, other than the tradition of writing on the welfare state from a comparative or Marxist perspective, requires us to think otherwise.

Nor, contrary to the view of Frances Piven and Richard Cloward, does the welfare state represent a mechanism to quiet workers at a time of discontent and put them in a "politically quiescent mode," to use political scientist Charles Lockhart's phrase. The American welfare state has experienced its greatest growth in times of prosperity. The welfare state does not constitute some sort of bribe to

keep sullen workers or members of racial minorities happy. If anything, money spent on social welfare programs only encourages further discontent and more demands for program expansion. Furthermore, most of the money gets spent in ways that make it difficult
to expand or contract expenditures according to the needs of the
labor market—if it even makes sense to talk of the labor market's
needs.

Neither simple view works for America. We need a different understanding of what drives public policy. I submit that policy often
reflects only itself. It stems from no grass-roots or large-scale demands. Programs get created for many complicated and particular
reasons—the very things that historians know how to unravel—and
then take on lives of their own. Nothing so influences policy debates
as previous policies. Ann Orloff, a sociologist who writes on the welfare
state, adds substance to this simple idea: "Policy debates are regularly
informed by ideas about how best to correct the perceived imper-
fections of past policy, rather than simply how to respond to social
conditions as such." In a similar sense, the politics of the welfare
state concerns tangible programs. Martha Derthick, a distinguished
political scientist, notes that policymaking and program extensions
have a "continuity, momentum, and political logic all their own."
Political scientist Theodore Lowi puts the matter even more bluntly.
"Policy," he says, "determines politics."

In thinking about the development of the welfare state from conflict
to consensus and back again, I emphasize four things about the
political process and American history. First, we did not set out in
1935 to create unpopular and unsuccessful programs. The programs
of the Social Security Act reflected the conventional wisdom of the
social insurance theorists whom President Roosevelt asked to write
the legislation. They believed, for example, that helping widows stay
home with their children was an idea beyond controversy. They
devoted far more attention to social insurance than to welfare because
they knew that social insurance posed many more political and economic problems.

Second, things did not work out as planned. The experts failed to
anticipate major changes in American life, such as an extraordinary
rise in the birth rate after the Second World War, a revolution in the
working patterns of women, and an exodus of blacks from the South
to the North. Each of these things changed the outlook of the people
who wanted to influence the policy process; but the program structures, once in place, proved remarkably resistant to change.

Third, many of the unforeseen events strengthened rather than undermined America's acceptance of the welfare state. Prosperity and a higher birth rate, for example, helped to nurture the growth of the Social Security program.

Fourth, the current attack on welfare does not constitute a full-scale assault on the American welfare state. Here the distinction between social insurance and welfare becomes important. Social insurance has two important characteristics. People who receive its benefits pay for at least some of those benefits themselves, or, alternatively, employers make contributions on behalf of their employees. People claim social insurance benefits as a matter of right, an entitlement. Welfare differs from social insurance on both counts. Its benefits come from general revenues and require no prepayment. Accepting welfare as a gratuity, people must prove to the state's satisfaction that they meet the entry conditions, such as having a dependent child in their care. Social Security constitutes our major form of social insurance, Aid to Families with Dependent Children (AFDC) our major form of welfare. Conservative critics have attacked welfare far more than social insurance.

Such criticisms reverse the priorities of the American welfare state. We spend far more on social insurance than on welfare, yet one would hardly know that from the constant criticisms directed at welfare. David Ellwood has assembled some telling statistics on this point. Correcting for inflation by using constant (1984) dollars, he estimates that we spent 55.1 billion on Social Security and 16.2 billion on basic welfare programs in 1960. Social Security's lead has increased over time. By 1984, we spent 242.8 billion on social security and 56.7 billion on welfare; and welfare benefits have grown very slowly since 1976, while Social Security benefits have continued their rapid expansion. Somehow the criticism of welfare does not quite match this statistical reality.

Even Social Security, although an enduring and popular program, has not escaped the recent criticism made of the American welfare state. The fact remains that we face a crisis in the welfare state in which once popular programs receive considerable scrutiny. This book marks an inquiry into that crisis, hoping to explain the cycle of controversy to consensus and back again by integrating the inner world of the policy process and the outer world of American history and culture.

Having explained the book's objectives, I should also delineate its self-conscious shortcomings. Three relatively brief case studies do not constitute an exhaustive study of the modern American welfare state. Neglected topics include food stamps, the role of business and labor in social welfare policy, the importance of federalism, and the role of public works programs such as the WPA (Works Progress Administration) or CETA (Comprehensive Employment and Training Act). I am sure that readers will notice other omissions. Furthermore, the book focuses on the policy process, primarily as perceived from within the bureaucracy. It concentrates on designing, approving, and administering government programs and neglects the realities underlying those programs, such as the experience of receiving social welfare benefits. It is not a social history of community action, welfare recipients, or the elderly.

More importantly, the book gives short shrift to three other important questions about the welfare state, to which I can suggest only tentative answers here. One concerns the tangible accomplishments of the welfare state. Some numbers help. Social Security has reduced the poverty rate, defined in 1988 as an income of $5,672 for a single individual over 65, from 35.2 percent of the elderly in 1959 to 12.2 percent in 1987. Forty-four percent of the elderly's income came from Social Security in 1987, and 47.5 percent of the elderly would have fallen below the poverty line in 1986 were it not for Social Security and other welfare benefits.

Another question involves the failures of the welfare state. These can be stated directly. Our social welfare programs have failed to stem the rise in single-parent families, failed to provide universal access to health care, failed to lift 15 percent of the population above the poverty line in 1983.

Finally, how do welfare recipients blend formal programs and informal sources of support? The answer to this question awaits the proper integration of policy studies and social history.

Each of the neglected subjects and the only partially answered questions deserves further consideration. For now, I ask the reader to accept this brief overview as useful in its own terms and to consider it as part of an ongoing exploration of America's welfare state that I began in 1980 with the publication of *Creating the Welfare State* and continued with books on disability policy (1987) and on a specific health care provider within the welfare state (1988). I hope to conclude with a biography of Wilbur Cohen, a central figure in the creation of the American welfare state.

Acknowledgments

Even authors of modest monographs acquire immodest debts. This book began when Bill Becker, the chair of my department, brought my name to Henry Tom's and Stanley Kutler's attention and suggested that I write for the Hopkins Press's American Moment Series. In the fullness of academic time, we reached an agreement and, as I settled down to do the research and writing, I received a fellowship from the Robert Wood Johnson Foundation to study health care finance. The fellowship enabled me to spend half a year at the Johns Hopkins Medical Institutions and half a year divided between the Health Insurance Association of America and the National Academy of Social Insurance. That gave me time to think about the American approach to health insurance, aided greatly by the suggestions of Vanessa Gamble, Carl Schramm, Charles Eby, Lucia Hatch, and John Gabel. Chapter 7, a preliminary version of which I delivered at the American Historical Association in December 1987, through the courtesy of Donald Critchlow, reflects those thoughts. Pamela Larson and Sara Berman, at the National Academy, supplied me with the congressional documents that I used to write Chapters 2 and 3. Robert Ball, also at the National Academy, generously allowed me access to his private memoranda on the 1983 Social Security amendments, and the Academy kept me well supplied with newspaper clippings concerning Social Security. The Twentieth Century Fund financed a trip to Minneapolis that gave me a chance to consult some of the collections at the Social Welfare History Archives. I am very grateful for the assistance of Clarke Chambers and David Klaasen. In addition, Blanche Coll permitted me to see advance chapters of her history of welfare, and that made it much easier to write Chapter 5. Frank Hubbard installed the computer on which I wrote most of this book. Wendy Wolff helped me to clarify my thoughts about health insurance.

Once drafts of the book reached the Johns Hopkins University Press, I received extraordinary help from Henry Tom, Stanley Kutler, and Mark Leff, each of whom commented on the typescript and made many helpful suggestions. Mark, in particular, has supported my scholarly efforts with the proper mixture of concern and enthusiasm. At the Press, Anne Whitmore edited the manuscript with precision and care.

Writing this book coincided with a period of transition in my job. Bill Becker and Leo Ribuffo, wonderful colleagues to whom I owe a great deal, helped me through the process. Many other historians went out of their way to support me and my work, and I thank each of them for their efforts. I also owe a continuing debt of gratitude to Kim McQuaid, who unfailingly supports my work.

This book also coincided with a creative collaboration with Eric Kingson, parts of which are reflected in Chapters 2, 3, and 4. Eric generously included me in the Nelson Cruikshank Study Project of the Save Our Security Educational Fund, from which I took much more than I gave.

At home I could not have completed the book without the help and support of my family, including Rebecca Alice Berkowitz, and of the members of my extended family. But, above all, this book is for my parents.

America's Welfare State

1   Introduction

By the end of the 1980s, America's social welfare programs had reached a state of crisis. The approaches put in place during the 1930s no longer seemed to be working, and the political situation offered no easy means of coming up with new approaches. The nation had backed itself into a corner, in part because the programs of the New Deal developed in unexpected ways. At first, they succeeded far beyond anyone's expectations. Then the situation began to deteriorate. As the programs came apart in the 1970s and 1980s, the nation never had a chance, in effect, to regroup and remake the system. The very presence of the old programs complicated the process of change. Vested bureaucratic and congressional interests blocked reform.

The welfare state is as old as America itself. When the first colonialists came to America, they brought welfare with them, and welfare continued to be a public concern after the country declared its independence from Britain. As states joined the union, they passed welfare laws. In a manner typical of such laws, the original Wisconsin legislation dealing with the care of the poor, passed in 1849 and closely modeled on similar laws in Pennsylvania, Ohio, and Michigan, stated broadly, "Every town shall relieve and support all poor and indigent persons, lawfully settled therein, whenever they shall stand in need thereof." Things seldom worked out as neatly as such sweeping statements implied. The welfare system remained profoundly local, and gaining welfare depended on satisfying the local authorities of real need and, above all, on being a legal resident who was "lawfully settled." Indigent strangers received warnings to leave town. Those who remained behind placed themselves at the mercy of the community, forced to accept whatever the community deemed appropriate: foster care, institutional confinement, compulsory work, or a cash grant.

In 1935, America took a different approach toward welfare and augmented its welfare state with "social security." The Social Security Act, the foundation on which modern social welfare policy rests, established the beginnings of the old-age insurance program that most people refer to as "Social Security." Nearly all of today's paystubs list a Social Security deduction. Functioning as a withholding tax that takes money from workers and uses that money to pay retirement pensions to the elderly and disabled, Social Security links the present state of employment with the future state of dependence.

We tend to forget that the 1935 act also marks the beginnings of national unemployment compensation and welfare. People laid off from their jobs who "go on unemployment" owe their benefits to a feature of the Social Security Act. The broad legislation also authorizes the federal government to pay the states and localities for welfare benefits for needy children, the elderly, and the blind.

The history of the Social Security Act from 1935 to the present underscores differences between outcomes and expectations. It demonstrates that history alters the plans of policymakers. Examples abound of how unforeseen events have obscured program origins and distorted initial goals. Social Security, welfare, and health insurance all conform to this general pattern. Although old-age insurance has become America's largest and most popular social welfare program, it began in far different circumstances. Although welfare now features many components designed to endow people with skills and remove them from the welfare rolls, this rehabilitation approach differs from the intentions of the people who created the program. Similarly, our system of national health insurance has developed in ways that few could have foreseen when the Social Security Act was written in 1935.

When the Social Security retirement program began, it reflected neither the will of Congress nor that of the people. If people had been free to choose, they would have chosen a program that gave every old person a pension, rather than one that excluded many workers, paid low benefits, and required workers to wait a minimum of five years before they could begin to receive pensions. Yet, at the urging of President Roosevelt, Congress made a less popular choice.

Social Security remained an insignificant program well into the 1940s, and it did not work as intended. Designed to be removed from partisan political control, the old-age insurance program became intensely political. Viewed as permanent rather than as emergency or temporary legislation, the program nonetheless required a major legislative overhaul within four years of its creation. Intended, above all, as a financially secure program that would never be in danger of going bankrupt, Social Security eventually developed severe financing problems that undermined people's faith in the program and required a major rescue operation. Even this rescue operation failed to save the program from controversy.

Because few people understood how Social Security really worked, the crises in Social Security appeared to come from nowhere. Some regarded Social Security as a simple savings bank with an automatic deposit feature. A person worked, made Social Security contributions, and then claimed his Social Security benefits at retirement. Barring catastrophically poor investments by the government, the system would function automatically and eliminate almost any chance of failure. By definition, a person received only benefits for which he had paid. Twice in recent years, however, this seamless system nearly ground to a halt, and people, particularly young people, began to doubt the system's financial integrity. Confidence quickly gave way to crisis. In 1977, for example, only 12 percent of the sample in a national poll believed that the Social Security system was financially sound. Seventy-five percent of the people aged 25–34 polled in June 1981 by CBS News and the *New York Times* doubted that Social security would provide full benefits for them. Behind such fears lay an emerging realization that Social Security was much more complicated than a savings bank; yet few Americans, even educated Americans, knew exactly where their money went.

As people pondered Social Security's future, welfare continued to be an unpopular alternative to social insurance. Contrary to its present reputation, welfare, in its post-1935 form, began as a popular, uncontroversial program that was run on a bipartisan basis. People clamored for more welfare benefits, rather than fewer, and not many people worried that welfare recipients were somehow exploiting the system to their advantage. Well into the 1950s, the typical welfare grant went to an old person who had worked his entire lifetime and now sought relief, rather than to a mother and her illegitimate child. Authorities expected welfare mothers to remain home and raise their children, not rehabilitate themselves and get a job. Far more white women received welfare than did black women.

Each of these things had changed by 1962. Within a few years, as attempts to rehabilitate welfare recipients brought only frustration, welfare became an unpopular, highly controversial program, populated by "chiselers." The typical welfare family now contained black children living in a house where the father was not present. Many recipients resided in cities, such as Baltimore, Detroit, Gary, Newark, and Washington, where, by 1980, a majority of residents were black. In March 1979, whites constituted only about half of the people on Aid to Families with Dependent Children (AFDC), and blacks made up nearly 44 percent of the caseload, although less than 12 percent of the general population was black. Many people came to see welfare dependency as a distinctively black problem, and the notion of putting black mothers to work, rehabilitating them from a life of welfare dependency, became popular.

Health insurance also developed in unforeseen ways. At first, authorities conceived of national health insurance as a program covering people of all ages. As it came into existence, in 1965, it covered only the elderly and those on welfare. Originally intended as a way of keeping costs within reasonable limits, national health insurance instead served as an important cause of health care cost inflation. By 1989, the nation's health care financing system lacked coherence. Most workers depended on their employers to pay the bulk of their medical bills, and most retirees relied on the financial generosity of the government to finance doctor visits and hospital stays. An alarming number of people, however, lacked any form of health insurance. When they went to the hospital, they hoped that the hospital or the community would pick up the tab.

The sense of crisis in Social Security, welfare, and health insurance marked the end of an optimistic era in which many people believed that the nation had solved, or would soon solve, its social welfare problems. This optimism found its expression in a belief that, with the right amount of government investment and expertise, the nation could eliminate poverty. In this century, two new methods of providing public welfare pointed the way toward the solution of social welfare problems. Social insurance marked the first new approach to public welfare. In the middle of the century, rehabilitation joined social insurance as a tool at the government's disposal in the fight against what experts referred to as "welfare dependency." Despite the development of these new approaches, things worked out differently. In the 1970s, optimism declined; poverty and problems persisted.

A major undertaking whose cost eventually amounted to one-tenth of the gross national product, social insurance took the form of a contract between the government and America's workers. Workers received protection against injury on the job and other forms of disability. They also benefited from a life insurance contract that covered their survivors. Most importantly, workers participated in a retirement program that included health insurance.

Such comprehensive coverage cost a great deal. In mid-1989, for example, 38.9 million Americans received some form of Social Security benefit. More Americans cashed checks from Social Security than lived in the entire country, North and South, during the Civil War. The Social Security beneficiary rolls contained more Americans than lived in any single state. Social Security benefits cost $236 billion a year; and to meet the costs, 131 million workers, and their employers, contributed about $250 billion into a special Social Security fund. Someone making $4,577 a month found $344 deducted for Social Security, the largest deduction from the check, with the exception only of the federal income tax. And these figures do not include all of America's social insurance programs. Expenditures for all social insurance programs in 1983 amounted to $330.6 billion.

The Social Security program reached more people than any other social program in American history, in part because it often sent checks to people who were neither poor nor needy, as a typical case from the files demonstrates. It concerns a New Jersey resident, born in 1919, who worked throughout his lifetime and paid Social Security taxes (which began in 1937) throughout his career. Toward the end of his career, his income became substantial, often exceeding $100,000 a year. In 1989, with no intention of retiring, he reached the age of 70, and the Social Security checks began arriving in the mail. Although he had no real need of the checks, they came anyway.

Beyond the sheer factors of scope and size, social insurance differed from the traditional "poor laws," as exemplified in the nineteenth-century Wisconsin law, in four ways. Where poor laws were administered by the localities, social insurance laws became the concern of federal and state governments. Where poor laws concentrated their aid on people who could demonstrate that they were poor, social insurance limited benefits to families headed by someone who had once worked. Where towns funded poor laws from revenues gathered through such means as property taxes, workers or their employers paid for social insurance themselves. Where the poor laws provided aid in many different forms, including lodging, food, and money, social insurance programs nearly always supplied beneficiaries with a check, the commodity they most wanted.

Viewed more broadly, the differences between the poor laws and social insurance reflect more general differences between nineteenth- and twentieth-century social policy. Nineteenth-century social policy made entitlement to public aid a function of location. If a person lived in a particular place for a certain period of time, he became the responsibility of that community. If his financial circumstances fell below a level that the community considered acceptable, then the community came to his aid. Twentieth-century social policy based entitlement to Social Security, the predominant form of public aid, on occupation. By working for a particular employer, an employee received the benefits of an insurance policy that protected him against situations that might interrupt his income.

In theory, social insurance represented a reorientation of the nation's welfare laws that was so sweeping as to render the older poor laws unnecessary. In reality, the old poor laws remained important, even in the late twentieth century. Welfare persisted because social insurance failed to cover all the contingencies that threatened people's financial security and because social insurance reached only families with an attachment to the labor force.

The statement of the problem suggested a remedy: expand social insurance coverage and devise a means to transform people so that they could participate in the labor force. In the postwar age of consensus, policymakers placed great credence on this grand design for social policy. In the era of crisis, neither of these solutions appeared to be within reach.

Social insurance covered many of the contingencies—industrial accident, unemployment, ill health, disability, and old age—that might stop a breadwinner from working. If, for example, a person's company suddenly went out of business, he could explain his situation at the local employment security office and promptly receive an unemployment check to tide him over while he searched for a new job. If the person reached the age of 65 and wanted to retire, he could expect monthly checks from Social Security.

At the same time, social insurance contained two significant gaps. In 1985, for example, some 35 million Americans lacked any form of health insurance. Nearly three-quarters of these uninsured people worked either full or part time or belonged to families in which someone worked.

Long-term care represented another serious omission. Suppose that someone retired at age 65 on Social Security and then became impaired to the point of needing to enter a nursing home. Social insurance would cover his visits to the doctor and his stays in the hospital. With very few exceptions, however, the system would force the person to pay for the nursing home out of his own pocket. If he or his family could not come up with the funds, the person faced no other choice but to depend on welfare.

Few people relished the thought of entering a nursing home. Indeed, such homes became the twentieth-century equivalents of a dreaded nineteenth-century institution: the poorhouse. For an old person, entering a nursing home signaled that he could no longer care for himself, that he required the nursing home's intrusive care in completing what the authorities in the field euphemistically called the "activities of daily living," such as getting dressed or using the toilet. The decision to enter a nursing home also carried the stigma of family failure. It implied a weakening of the family bond in a time of crisis, since the person's children could not or simply would not put up mom or dad at home. Rich people hired personal attendants or entered a fashionable retirement community. People who did not have that kind of money went to a nursing home, spent all of their assets, and then relied on the state government to pay the tab until they died. Because the social insurance system did not cover long-term care, the welfare system picked up the slack.

Not only did the twentieth-century social insurance system not handle all of modern life's emergencies, it also did not cover the entire American population. Faced with a catastrophic situation, many people fell back on welfare. Nearly 11 million mothers and children, more people than the combined populations of New York, Chicago, and Baltimore, received welfare in 1984.

It was in 1985 that Maeola Drakeford's daughter joined the rolls. One day Maeola Drakeford came to work looking disappointed. Her daughter, it seemed, was pregnant. For Maeola, a deeply religious woman, abortion lay beyond the realm of possibility, and that meant that the daughter, who accepted her mother's authority, would bring the baby to term. In all likelihood, the daughter would be allowed to complete her senior year of high school and graduate, but the school had a strict policy of not allowing girls who were "showing" to take part in the graduation ceremonies. That proved a source of deep disappointment to Maeola.

No men lived in the house, and neither Maeola nor her daughter earned much money. Maeola's husband had long since left the scene. The father of the daughter's baby refused to acknowledge his responsibility toward the daughter or the baby she was carrying; that meant Maeola and her daughter faced the situation by themselves. They already received some public assistance in the form of subsidized housing, but, with the arrival of the new baby, they would require more money. They would have to visit the local social service office and ask for what Maeola, with her soft southern accent, called "hep." In all likelihood, the local social service office would supply that help by putting Maeola's daughter and her new grandchild on welfare. Maeola and her daughter hoped that the new baby would be a girl, both because they believed that a girl would be easier to manage in a household where child care arrangements would be makeshift and because they knew that a girl would herself be able

---

to go on welfare should she someday get in trouble and require "hep." Here, then, was a black baby born in public housing in the inner city and dependent, from its very first minutes on this earth, on welfare.

Social statistics indicate that Maeola's daughter's situation was not unusual. In 1980, for example, well over half of all black births occurred outside of marriage. Most black children lived in one-parent families. In 1984, over 89 percent of the births among black women aged 15–19 were illegitimate.

To cope with such complicated matters as mothers who bore children out of wedlock and failed to develop a permanent connection with the labor force, policymakers devised rehabilitation. The rehabilitation approach suggested that Maeola's daughter might be transferred from a state of welfare dependency to a position of self-sufficiency. Learning a skill, for example, might lead to a job. Beyond the world of welfare lay the reassurances of the world of work, including social insurance protection against life's major hazards. Although mother and baby continued to collect welfare as the rehabilitation process unfolded, the welfare payments served only as a temporary way station while Maeola's daughter gathered the opportunities, skills, and courage to face working.

Rehabilitation, a modern innovation, supplemented three older approaches to welfare, including prevention, deterrence, and maintenance. The same tradition that mandated communities to take care of the poor also included precepts related to preventing social problems. As an example, the common law that America inherited from England required employers to take "reasonable care" to prevent injuries in the workplace and to pay damages to their injured employees. In effect, the threat of a law suit deterred employers from exposing employees to dangerous conditions and helped to prevent accidents.

Deterrence, as applied to workers rather than employers, constituted a harsher approach than prevention. The poorhouse emerged as the symbol of this approach. In 1824, for example, the New York state legislature formed a committee to investigate rising welfare costs. The committee recommended the construction of poorhouses in each county. With rising rates of immigration, some of the local poorhouses became designated as special places for paupers who, because they lacked a permanent settlement in any town, became the state's responsibility. By the end of the nineteenth century, New York's poorhouses served a substantial number of people. Michael Katz estimates that in 1900 the state's local and county poorhouses supported as many as 85,500 people.

Many poorhouse residents fell into a nebulous category of people who were neither lazy nor able to find work. By the middle of the nineteenth century, such people found themselves subjected to increasingly sophisticated tests designed to deter "malingerers" from accepting the community's hospitality. As developed in England by Edwin Chadwick and other Victorian social policy experts, the poorhouse provided a level of comfort that was pegged, at least in theory, to the exact level of subsistence. If it took eighty calories for a man to survive, the poorhouse diet supplied eighty-one. According to Chadwick's theory, only people who truly needed aid would agree to live under such conditions. For others the threat of the poorhouse served as a prod that deterred them from idleness.

Although some cities, such as Brooklyn in the 1870s, temporarily suspended grants of food and coal or "outdoor relief," such grants and their implicit policy of maintaining the poor at public expense remained a public welfare staple. In the first place, many of the poor, such as the indigent blind, suffered from conditions serious enough to excuse them from working. Nineteenth-century authorities believed it appropriate, therefore, for such people to depend on the community for maintenance. In New York, the state legislators made repeated attempts to remove various members of the "deserving poor," such as insane people and children, from poorhouses. In the second place, "outdoor relief," often easier and more politically rewarding to administer than a poorhouse, provided short-term help for the hungry or homeless, whatever the contemporary theory for the proper conduct of social policy. Still, as Katz notes, America continued to provide welfare "in the shadow of the poorhouse."

Rehabilitation, by way of contrast, reflected a twentieth-century optimistic sense that threats were no longer so necessary, that nearly anyone who wanted to participate in the national economy could do so, and that technology could overcome physical or mental problems. Where the poorhouse and other nineteenth-century institutions relied on a strategy of segregation—removing people from their families and from their communities—rehabilitation as an approach to social policy depended on integration. Rehabilitation encouraged welfare mothers to join the economic mainstream. It exposed the residents of black ghettos to the wider world around them. It removed people with disabilities from asylums and placed them in regular schools.

Behind the optimism of the rehabilitation approach and its strategy of integration lay a revolution in labor force expectations. In the nineteenth century, authorities conceded many groups a safe haven outside of the labor force. Most women, for example, did not work outside of the home; in the twentieth century, women's participation in the labor force became the norm. In 1975, for the first time in American history, a majority of the nation's mothers with school-age children held jobs outside of the home. The expectation that most women would participate in the labor force gradually came to apply to women on welfare as well. As late as 1935, policymakers believed it important for mothers to stay home and take care of their children. They even encouraged the use of public money for that purpose, should the father die and leave the mother in financial difficulties. In time, however, policymakers began to expect people like Maeola's daughter to work. She could no longer benefit from prevention; she required neither maintenance nor deterrence but rather rehabilitation.

In the twentieth century, social insurance and rehabilitation have come to define our approach to social welfare policy. At first, each of these approaches struggled against a sense that they increased government power beyond accepted bounds and offered little in the way of practical results. Then, by mid-century, American policymakers accepted them as mechanisms that promised to solve enduring social welfare problems and illustrated the pragmatic way in which America blended public and private power. Finally, in the 1970s and 1980s, rehabilitation and social insurance became identified as sources of, rather than solutions to, social problems, and as agents responsible for the crisis of the welfare state. Unfortunately, policymakers came up with little to offer in their place.

Introduction

★ ★ ★

I

The Social Security Crisis

Inventing Social Security, 1935

President Roosevelt approached Social Security, the cornerstone of the American welfare state, with a sense of leisure that belied the economic crisis facing the country. For well over a year, other items, such as trying to bring the economy out of the severest depression in the nation's history and meeting the demand for food and shelter, had prior claims on the president's attention. As Roosevelt's deliberate and measured attitude toward the legislation suggested, Social Security did not represent a response to the country's immediate problems so much as an attempt to reform conditions in the labor market. When the Social Security Act became law, in August 1935, it permanently altered the terms of employment by requiring employers and employees to participate in a retirement program run by the federal government and making it mandatory for an employer to pay money to employees, even after they had been laid off. The president's supporters believed that these new programs provided the employee with some security against what Roosevelt called the "hazards and vicissitudes of life."

Far-reaching as these measures were, they met with less than total approval from workers, politicians, and others who felt that the government should fight the present depression before undertaking to prevent the next one. Economic conditions, desperate in 1933 when Roosevelt took office, remained bleak in 1935. Although the New Deal programs instituted in the spring of 1933 produced some improvement, the best guesses put the 1935 unemployment rate at about 20 percent, meaning that about one out of every five persons still in the labor force did not have a job. Others—no one knew just how many—

had lost hope and stopped looking for work. The high unemployment rate indicated that many of the nation's plants, factories, and stores lay idle or abandoned, as though someone had decided not to use all of America's productive capacity. Misery and despair remained, even though fewer people sold apples on the street corners than in 1933 and fewer people lived in make-shift shanty towns, known as Hoovervilles in honor of Roosevelt's predecessor, such as the one in Oklahoma City that covered 100 square miles and contained people squatting in what one eyewitness remembered as "old, rusted out car bodies," orange crates, and holes in the ground.

Of all the components of the Social Security Act, old-age insurance, the program that would ultimately become the most successful and popular, received the harshest criticism. Republicans, who went along with giving money to the unemployed, called old-age insurance, in the words of the ranking member of the House Ways and Means Committee, "the worst title in the bill . . . a burdensome tax on industry, a compulsory, arbitrary program." "Nobody is going to get a dime out of this until 1942," another Republican complained, "This will not buy bread for anybody now." Liberal congressmen grumbled that there would be "bitter disappointment." Local politicians reacted in a similar manner, the Mayor of Baltimore calling the entire Social Security Act "the most asinine thing I have ever read in my life."

Despite the persistent criticism, President Roosevelt proposed this politically unappealing program and insisted that it become law. His reasons centered on his deep desire to remove the federal government from the provision of cash grants to able-bodied individuals. In this respect, he made a sharp differentiation between welfare, which paid people for doing nothing, and social insurance, which rewarded people for working. Welfare, said Roosevelt, operated like a "narcotic, a subtle destroyer of the human spirit"; social insurance, in the president's view, constituted a "sound means" of providing economic security. To establish social insurance, Roosevelt resolved to spend some of the political capital that had accrued over the first two years of his term and push for legislation that he knew would bring negligible political rewards.

Ironically, President Roosevelt owed much of his political popularity to his willingness to dispense with moral scruples and endorse emergency relief spending. In the first giddy days of the administration, he had taken steps to shore up the nation's faltering welfare system. By May 12, 1933, Congress had authorized half a billion dollars in relief. Harry Hopkins, a social worker and former New York State colleague of Roosevelt's who was placed in charge of the hastily created Federal Emergency Relief Agency, worked with local officials

The Social Security Crisis

across the nation to keep people from starving. By March 1934, an unprecedented number of citizens were receiving welfare, financed largely by federal funds but distributed by local authorities. In that month, for example, the welfare rolls in Baltimore reached 64,876 cases, well over 30 percent of the city's population.

Massive relief of this sort made President Roosevelt uneasy. He had no intention of replacing the traditional poor law system with federal funds. If it was necessary for the government to provide relief, Roosevelt believed it should take the form of jobs, rather than straight handouts. Accordingly, he proceeded with plans to launch a massive public works program that became part of the Emergency Relief Appropriations Act of 1935 and featured the establishment of the Works Progress Administration, universally known as the WPA.

Plans for Social Security moved along a different track. They fell under the rubric, in Roosevelt's words, of "rebuilding many of the structures of our economic life and reorganizing it in order to prevent a recurrence of collapse." Toward this end, he vowed in June 1934 to "further the security of the citizen and his family through social insurance" and announced that he was looking for a way "to provide at once against several of the disturbing factors in life—especially those that relate to unemployment and old age." In the next three weeks, Roosevelt established a cabinet-level committee, chaired by Secretary of Labor Frances Perkins, to formulate coherent recommendations. The staff of the Committee on Economic Security, under the direction of University of Wisconsin professor Edwin Witte, created Social Security in the summer and fall of 1934.

Congress responded warily, passing the law in the summer of 1935 as an act of prudent faith. It was prudent to side with Roosevelt, who, after all, had won a resounding vote of confidence in the 1934 congressional elections and made it possible for the Democrats to consolidate their hold over Congress. It was an act of faith to believe that the legislation would solve social problems. From all accounts, Congress understood little about the complex piece of legislation that it had received. In the end, the bill passed because President Roosevelt wanted it to pass.

Old-Age Insurance: Past Precedents and Future Hopes

Neither the president nor Congress designed old-age insurance; the task fell instead to three experts on the Committee on Economic Security staff, none of whom achieved fame or substantial recognition for their efforts. Two of the three were refugees from academia who wanted to assist President Roosevelt with the work of the New Deal.

Barbara Armstrong taught in the law school at the University of California, Berkeley, and Douglas Brown worked as an economist at Princeton University. Murray Latimer, the third member of the group, designed pension plans for large companies, the sort of person who carried mechanical pencils in his front pocket. These, then, were not politicians, concerned about winning the next election, but rather theoreticians or social policy experts, anxious to guide Frances Perkins, Franklin Roosevelt, and the members of Congress toward the right approach to the problems of old-age in America. Each of these creators tended to treat Social Security more as an academic exercise and less as a crash program to get money into the hands of the elderly at a time of economic catastrophe. The deliberations involved the subtleties of history, demography, and economics, not an ideological desire to harness workers' discontent and move America closer toward a welfare state.

The three experts plunged into their work in the summer of 1934. Doing what came naturally, they first defined their objective, to find a way for the federal government to raise the income of the elderly, and then studied existing programs and proposals. They discovered that in a majority of states people who were old and poor did not have to go a poorhouse or a similar institution but could instead claim cash pensions from the state government, rather than from the local welfare authorities. The experts soon found, however, that these state programs fell far short of solving the problems of the elderly, as the conditions they examined in Ohio demonstrated.

Ohio, like twenty-seven other states in 1935, ran an old-age pension program that came nowhere near to meeting the elderly's demand for welfare. In a population of 450,000 over the age of 65, more than 100,000 Ohio residents applied to the program. Approval of pensions took time because each application received intensive scrutiny. An elderly person applied to a county board, which exercised considerable discretion over who actually received a pension, because, as one knowledgeable person put it, the boardmembers "know pretty nearly everybody in the county and they can either refuse to approve, hold it up, make their own personal investigation." These boards employed investigators who issued reports on each applicant; and, even if the county board approved the pension, the application then went to state authorities who employed their own inspectors who made sure that the application met the terms of the law.

As the stringent terms of the Ohio law made clear, not everyone received an old-age pension. There was, first of all, a minimum eligible age of 65. There was a residence requirement of 15 years in the state of Ohio and one year in the same county. There were moral restrictions. Someone who neglected his children or had deserted his wife could be denied a pension, so could someone who had been convicted of drunkenness. The law limited the pensions to those who could prove poverty, requiring the applicant to affirm that his income was less than $300 a year and that the net value of his real estate did not exceed $4,000. Although proven poor and awarded a pension, a person could still lose his grant on moral grounds, such as by misspending or wasting the grant.

The grant of $50 a month for a married couple represented a loan to the elderly that was secured by a lien against their estate. If the couple owned a house worth more than $500, they had to turn the house over to the state of Ohio. They could continue living there for the rest of their lives; then the state had the right to sell the house and pocket the proceeds as recompense for the old-age pension. By 1935, after only ten months of the law's operation, the state had taken $2.5 million worth of property in trust. As the director of the program explained, "after the state gets its money, then come the next of kin, or whoever can qualify under the law, . . . but the state comes first." According to the director, complaints were few, in part because the recipients of the pensions had no "recourse in law at all . . . no right in court. It is purely a gratuity, in other words."

Not all elderly citizens in need of special assistance went through this demeaning process. Veterans of the nation's wars applied directly to the federal government for welfare, and in many cases received it. Where the states hedged their programs with excessive restrictions, the federal government awarded veterans pensions with a sense of abandon. The most notorious program, described in 1934 by President Roosevelt's advisors as a "raid on the treasury," covered Civil War veterans, their wives, and, in some cases, their children. It began modestly but grew into an entity that covered at least one-half of all elderly native-born men in the North and consumed a third of the federal budget in 1890.

Reviewing state and veterans' programs for the elderly, President Roosevelt's advisors, true to their academic outlook, searched for lessons and found two. One was that programs for the elderly needed to be strictly separated from partisan politics. Otherwise, politicians would use welfare as a means of rewarding their friends and punishing their enemies, and abuses would occur. The other was that, since expenditures on welfare for the elderly tended to grow over time, policymakers needed to find some way of anticipating and controlling future costs. Otherwise, Congress would blithely promise to pay benefits to people in the future without comprehending the cost of those benefits, placing huge burdens on unsuspecting future generations.

Simply put, the academicians distrusted the politicians and wanted to substitute expert administration for political discretion. Believing that politics was inherently antithetical to effective public administration, they filled their reports with sermons and exhortations on the need for sound administrative practices. Nothing, the staffmembers wrote, "is more important than personnel." Nothing would so greatly discredit the programs they hoped to create as would "poor administration, which inevitably results from the use of untrained, poorly qualified, politically appointed, and constantly shifting personnel." They strived for "uniformity of administrative effectiveness" and hoped to achieve it through a board, "protected as far as possible from political influence," staffed by "outstanding persons in the field of social insurance administration."

The experts believed that, unlike politicians, they knew how to delay gratification and how to consider the future consequences of present actions. Members of Congress, who lacked a similar sense of restraint, could be expected to seize on a temporary budget surplus as an excuse for expanding benefits to the elderly, aware only of the next election and unmindful of the commitment being made to younger people. When the future arrived, the nation could all too easily find itself saddled with unwanted debt. Experts, by way of contrast, possessed the necessary skills to calculate future costs and the vision to see beyond the next election.

Even as the president's advisors studied the past, they heard constant cries to initiate new programs for the elderly. If they failed to come up with an acceptable plan, they knew that others, eager to exploit the economic misery of the Depression for political advantage, stood ready and willing to offer plans of their own. Huey Long, the flamboyant senator from Louisiana, whom President Roosevelt regarded as one of the two most dangerous men in America, wanted to spend $3.6 billion to give anyone over age 60 a pension. Shrewdly playing on the nation's psychology in the middle of the deep depression, Long portrayed his program as a means of sharing "our" wealth; he wanted to return money to the poor that had been taken from them. To emphasize this point, he proposed to extract the funds for his pensions from a tax levied only on millionaires, because as one of Long's congressional allies put it, "you have to get down to the cream of the wealth, . . . down to the enormous fortunes and to the swollen, predatory wealth."

Another popular plan owed its name to Dr. Francis Townsend, a

California doctor who had devised a scheme to pay $200 a month to people over 60 years of age. Not everyone qualified; one had to be an American citizen, and the plan excluded convicted felons. Still, the plan contained few other qualifications, so that as many as 11 million people would receive pensions at an estimated cost of $2.4 billion. Unlike Long, Townsend favored a sales tax, rather than an income tax, as a means of financing the pensions.

The elderly responded enthusiastically to Townsend's plan when it appeared in 1934; the president's experts reacted with characteristic caution. As many as 25 million people signed petitions in support of the Townsend plan; across the nation, the elderly formed 1200 clubs to advance the Townsend cause. The experts analyzed the plan and decided that the numbers simply did not add up. They calculated that the proposed tax could support the program for only three months, because the costs of the benefits would amount to half of the nation's income. Secretary of Labor Frances Perkins called the Townsend plan, "a dole, a very large present . . . a very large gift . . . much larger than the income which they enjoyed during their younger and working years." Douglas Brown complained that the high sales taxes needed to fund the Townsend plan would "discourage business."

Dr. Townsend argued that Secretary Perkins and Professor Brown had missed the point. They had looked at the plan only as a pension plan, dismissing two important details. One was the requirement that pension recipients spend all of the money they received each month, and the other was that the elderly retire in order to get the pension. As Townsend put it, "this plan is only incidentally a pension plan. The old people are simply to be used as a means by which prosperity will be restored to all of us." Because the plan would put so much money into circulation, said Townsend, consumption would be "constantly raised to the level of our productive ability." Because the elderly would retire, young people would be in a position "to demand and receive decent wages." Townsend said that the president's advisors dismissed his plan precisely because it was so logical and so simple. "Every time a 'brain truster' says this plan is crazy, a hundred new converts come to our banner," he noted.

Brown, Armstrong, and Latimer, studying old and new programs, decided to create their own. They came up with a three-part system for alleviating the insecurities of old age. Part one consisted of a social insurance plan. Part two contained a new welfare program for the elderly. Part three involved a voluntary insurance policy sold by the government that people could purchase, much like a private insurance policy, at local post offices and banks.

Roosevelt's advisors regarded old-age insurance, their social insurance proposal, as a dignified alternative to the state pensions, such as the one in Ohio, that nonetheless would not bankrupt the government. Their plan would take the form of a guaranteed contract—an insurance policy—into which workers and their employers made regular contributions and from which they received regular monthly retirement benefits from the federal government beginning at age 65. No one who made regular contributions would be refused benefits, ending such practices as taking the family homestead as collateral payment for a retirement pension or forcing people to prove they were poor before they could collect a pension. The plan, in short, protected an individual's dignity. "It is contributory and contractual and affords an annuity as a matter of right," explained Douglas Brown.

As Brown's description implied, Brown, Armstrong, and Latimer rejected Townsend and Long's approach of simply giving the elderly money. They spurned what they called "gratuitous pensions," because they did not think the federal government could sustain such a program. Eventually, it would become too costly. The staff knew that, although there were 6.6 million Americans over 65 in 1930, they could expect that number to rise substantially by 1980. They thought there might be 17 million elderly then; and, as it turned out, that guess proved too conservative, since the actual number was closer to 25.5 million. A growing population of elderly citizens meant rising costs for old-age pensions. Hence, the planners made two fundamental assumptions. First, the costs would eventually become too great for the government to bear. Second, workers and employers should pay for their retirement pensions themselves, rather than relying on the government's general revenues. That provided a way of taking the costs of retirement pensions "off budget," to use the modern idiom. Through the adoption of social insurance, Edwin Witte explained, "the rapidly increasing cost of gratuitous pensions will, in the course of time, be greatly reduced."

The president's advisors chose a payroll tax as the suggested means of financing their social insurance proposal, even though they knew that such a tax penalized the poor, the very group who needed government help the most. If, for example, the government decided to tax all people's wages at a rate of 1 percent, then a bond holder who stayed home and clipped coupons would be taxed far more lightly than someone who worked in a factory and depended on every penny in his pay check.

Why, then, did the staff not recommend a broader-based tax, such as an income tax, that would have allowed some of the nation's "predatory" wealth to be spent on old-age pensions? The answer

The Social Security Crisis

concerned the state of public finance in 1934. In this era before the federal government learned how to withhold money from a worker's weekly paycheck, income tax rates remained very low, so low, in fact, that even if the rates had been increased, they still would not have provided enough money for Social Security pensions. As historian Mark Leff has noted, more than 95 percent of the public paid no income tax in 1935, and most of the rest made very small payments. Other alternatives, such as sales taxes, not only penalized low-income workers, who spent (rather than saved) more of their income than did higher-income workers, but also forced those not covered by old-age insurance to pay for pensions that they would never receive. The remaining alternative was payroll taxes, taking money directly out of the workers' paychecks.

Payroll taxes meshed nicely with the planners' desires to control political appetites. The taxes placed the emphasis where the planners thought it belonged: on the future. Workers participated in a contractual relationship that would yield future benefits. That meant that Congress could not arbitrarily cut the benefits for which people had, in a sense, paid, nor, it was hoped, could they raise the benefits much beyond the ability of workers and employers to finance them. The planners, then, saw the payroll taxes as a way of short-circuiting the greedy, pork-barrel behavior they expected from Congress.

Although taxing payrolls appeared to be a sensible, if conservative, way to finance retirement pensions in America's fledgling welfare state, the approach failed to eliminate problems related to the rising costs of the pensions. Here the tyranny of economics and the nature of the planners' rules took over.

Under these rules, not everyone received a pension. It was necessary to put some money into the system to get anything back. Social insurance always operated under this type of restriction; you had to pay to play. When the old-age insurance program started, therefore, it would have low expenses and high revenues. Under the pay and play rule, no one would be eligible for a pension, keeping costs low, but many would be paying into the system, keeping revenues high. As time passed the situation would change; more and more people, who had contributed to the system, would retire. That would definitely raise costs without necessarily raising revenues. The number of people who retired, after all, had nothing to do with the number of people who were working and paying taxes. Here was a true dilemma: raising enough money to cover costs, easy in the beginning, would become harder and harder as time passed and more and more people retired.

How should the old-age insurance program deal with this iron law of rising costs? One possible means relied on matching revenues and expenses each year. Actuaries could calculate the bill for each year and then set the payroll taxes at the right levels to pay the bill. This idea, although simple and practical, contained the hidden flaw of discriminating against young people. If each year the program collected only enough money to pay current operating costs, then older people would receive a real bargain. In all likelihood, they would pay less and receive more. Although the pay and play rule required them to make at least some contributions, these contributions would be relatively small, because initial program expenses would be so low. After only a few years of making contributions, they would themselves retire and begin receiving benefits. Young people faced the prospect of contributing during their entire working lifetime and paying higher and higher taxes as the costs of the system rose over time. In this manner, younger people ended up paying the bill for older people who had contributed little to the system.

As an example, someone 60 years old in 1937 might pay a 1 percent tax for 5 years and then retire. Someone who was 20 years old in 1937 might pay a 1 percent tax for 5 years, followed by a higher tax for the next 40 years.

The planners liked nothing better than this sort of demographic challenge. By making a few calculations, they saw the impossibility of pay-as-you-go, and so they looked for ways of evening the burden across generations. But they kept running into the difficulties imposed by their own rules for a contributory, self-sustaining system, run on a nonpartisan basis. Only two alternatives to a pay-as-you-go system existed, and both contained flaws. One involved using general tax revenues, but that meant abandoning the notion that people paid for their pensions. Another consisted of collecting money in advance as a way of meeting future costs, but that meant running surpluses in the early years of the program. Planners worried about how Congress would administer those surplus funds at a time of budget deficits and constant demands for spending to meet the urgent problems of the Depression. Could one part of the budget be in surplus if the overall budget was in deficit?

Brown, Armstrong, and Latimer eventually arrived at a solution that they regarded as sensible and even-handed. They proposed a gradually rising tax rate, split evenly between the employer and the employee, that would begin in 1937 at 2 percent and rise every 2 years until it reached 5 percent in 1957. At first, the program would have a bit too much money, but in time it would collect a bit too little. A deficit would develop by about 1967. When that year arrived, Brown and his associates felt, instead of raising the tax rate above 5 percent, the federal government should make up the deficit with general revenues. They argued that by 1967 the system and the principle of contributory, rather than "free," pensions would be well-established. It made sense for the government to subsidize old-age insurance, just as foreign governments did.

At this point the academic experts came into conflict with the politicians. President Roosevelt, who liked so much else about the plan, dismissed the financing proposal as immoral and politically naive. A fiscal conservative, Roosevelt felt that his advisors were recommending that he impose a debt on future generations. In 1967, current taxpayers would have to pay for pensions that should have been financed through payroll tax collections. Roosevelt, in other words, wanted old-age insurance to be completely self-supporting. All of the money for the program would have to come from payroll taxes, none from general revenues.

When Roosevelt discovered the "government subsidy" in the plan, in January 1935, he summoned staff director Edwin Witte to the White House. In Witte's presence, Roosevelt crossed out the word "subsidy" from the draft report, replaced the word with "deficit," and told Witte to rework the tax rates. Secretary of the Treasury Henry Morgenthau and the Committee on Economic Security staff came up with a new plan that met Roosevelt's wishes by raising the tax rate to 6 percent as early as 1949. At these rates, there would be no deficit, and the old-age insurance program would never have to draw on general revenues. Money raised from employers and employees would take care of all its needs. By the same token, however, that meant that for many years, the system would collect far more money than it would spend.

The politics of old-age pensions in early 1935 presented a study in stark contrasts. On one side stood President Roosevelt and his advisors, poring over charts that showed, on the basis of demographic and economic projections, a future deficit in a program that had not yet been proposed, much less passed into law and put into operation. Senator Long and Dr. Townsend, on the other side, wanted to put the government behind an absolute guarantee, now and for the future, to pay generous pensions to the elderly. The president pondered the morality of spending money from the federal budget in 1967 to pay for a program enacted in 1935; neither Long nor Townsend worried about the future or bothered to consult technical experts. These differences sharpened the suspicions of one side toward the other. Long and Townsend accused Roosevelt's advisors of neglecting present needs; Roosevelt's advisors denounced Long and Townsend for mortgaging the future.

Long and Townsend, stirring up popular support for old-age pensions, enjoyed the luxury of being able to present their plans in broad outline; the president's experts, in effect preparing the proposal of record, faced the unenviable task of anticipating future problems and attempting to solve them. Where Townsend could propose immediate pensions of $200 a month, Roosevelt's advisors, committed to the idea of social insurance, needed to worry about the relationship between a person's contributions and his benefits.

They realized that a self-financing *system,* on which the president insisted, bore little or no relationship to pensions that people paid for themselves. Roosevelt hoped to prevent the system from going into debt but raised no objections to allowing some people to subsidize the pension of others. As all parties to the dispute understood, older people needed pensions at least as badly as younger people, yet had fewer years to make contributions into the Social Security fund. That dilemma raised a simple question. Should older people be given "junk" pensions, based strictly on their contributions, or should the government establish a minimum level for the pensions? If someone were 60 years old when the plan began in 1937, earned a steady amount of $50 a month, made 5 years of contributions, and retired in 1942 at the agreed-upon retirement age of 65, he would have "earned," at the contemplated contribution rates, a pension of about 25¢ a month. The planners regarded that as too little. They substituted a minimum pension of $10 a month and a formula that gave low-income and older people a greater return on their contribution than higher-income and younger people. As Witte explained, people who are "now past middle age will not pay their own pensions entirely."

Even the president's prudent old-age insurance plan, therefore, followed complicated rules that went far beyond establishing a government savings bank and encouraging people to bank some of their pay check until they could retire and draw on their savings. Not everyone received the same rate of interest from the account that they and their employers were forced to open with the government. People with more money subsidized people with less money; younger people subsidized older people.

And some people never received anything; they were completely excluded. The plan called for tax collections to begin in 1937 and the first regular benefits to be paid in 1942. People who retired before 1937 were out of luck; those who left the labor force between 1937 and 1942 received only a lump-sum payment, reflecting their contributions plus interest. Almost all of these people faced the painful alternatives of making it on private savings or accepting welfare. Still others worked in occupations that were not covered by the proposed social insurance plan. They, too, would not receive a retirement pension as a guaranteed right but would either have to qualify for welfare, keep working until they died, or go it alone.

The three analysts advising Roosevelt tended to think of old-age insurance as something for industrial laborers who made less than $3,000 a year. It made administrative sense to collect a payroll tax from workers who maintained a stable relationship with a single employer. They decided to exclude a self-employed person, who was both employer and employee, from social insurance. Farm laborers and domestic servants were also excluded under the staff's proposal.

The staff characterized farm labor as an occupation in which "a large number of individual workers are employed in small establishments, frequently at some distance from any city or town." Unlike large industrial employers, farmers, according to a popular prejudice that the Social Security planners did not challenge, kept poor records of their payroll, and in many cases hired live-in help, which meant that part of the laborer's income took the form of room and board. All of that would hinder "effective enforcement" and led Brown and company to accept the advice of Abraham Epstein, a noted expert on social insurance, who said, "Start modestly. Do not try to collect now from the farmers."

Domestic servants, in a similar manner, suffered from the popular stereotype that they worked for many different employers, could not keep accurate records, and received many benefits, such as food and spare clothes, in kind. Planners, whether consciously or unconsciously, hesitated to burden housewives with the task of keeping records of their Social Security contributions on behalf of their domestic servants. Domestic servants joined farmers as excluded occupations.

Coverage limitations further obscured the already dim connection between social insurance and social need. Although the Social Security planners did not neglect the concept that some people were needier than others and required more help than others, they failed to address the problems of the nation's neediest citizens. Some old people received a subsidy; other people were considered too old to help. Some poor people received a subsidy; other people were regarded as, in effect, too far outside the regular labor force—too poor—to help. In the end, social insurance did not concern helping the needy, so much as providing a base of security for the nation's industrial population. It was not about the current depression so much as the next one.

Brown, Armstrong, and Latimer, who did not lack social compas-

140, 165

sion, buttressed their suggestions for social insurance with suggestions of more immediate importance to the nation's elderly citizens. Here the two other parts of their plan came into play. One part called for federal contributions to help state authorities grant pensions to the elderly. This part relied on welfare rather than social insurance. The other part consisted of special pensions that people not covered by social insurance could buy directly from the government. Together, the three parts constituted a well-rounded proposal, yet the advisors devoted most of their time and attention to social insurance, not welfare or what they called "voluntary annuities."

In January 1935, having completed their elaborate plans for old-age security, the advisors slipped back to the classroom, and Congress began consideration of the Economic Security Act. The process, long and tedious, consumed the winter and much of the spring of 1935. President Roosevelt signed the bill in August.

The bill that the planners left behind for Congress to consider contained few compromises and an astonishing number of political liabilities. Most of the congressmen represented agricultural districts, yet the bill contained little of direct benefit to farmers. Most of the congressmen received a surfeit of mail from supporters of the Townsend plan, yet the bill responded to the elderly in a far less generous way than did the Townsend plan. Most of the congressmen paid considerable deference to the employers in their districts, yet the bill imposed new payroll taxes on these employers and gave them no choice about paying them. The bill also threatened important special interests, such as insurance companies.

Congressional debate exposed each of these liabilities, yet the bill passed anyway. The planners represented Roosevelt, and the president, for reasons of his own, decided to fight for the legislation. The measure emerged from Congress virtually intact, but not without having received considerable criticism.

Congress neatly reversed the planners' priorities. Where the planners spent most of their time devising old-age insurance and threw in welfare as a way of rounding out the measure, the congressmen concentrated on the welfare features of the measure and generally ignored old-age insurance. Where the planners devoted considerable time to devising ways of meeting future contingencies, the congressmen limited their vision to the problems of the immediate present.

It was no accident, therefore, that welfare, rather than social insurance, appeared at the top of the bill, after lawyers from the Department of Labor and the Committee on Ways and Means worked over drafts prepared by the president's advisors. Welfare became Title I of the long legislation. No one, not a single congressman, spoke against the idea of federal grants to the states to pay old-age pensions to needy citizens. For every dollar that the states contributed, the federal government would chip in a dollar, up to a maximum of fifteen federal dollars per recipient per month. Even very conservative congressmen conceded the need for a "temporary contribution" in the "present emergency." Republicans joined liberal Democrats in arguing for higher pensions and greater federal contributions. One Democratic congressman, elected from a traditionally Republican district with considerable help from the Townsend movement, worried that the "college professors" had come to Washington and offered a "pauper's dole" to "God's beloved old people." The political issue was that the legislation involved not too much welfare, but rather too little.

Social insurance, which took second place to welfare in the bill, received little mention in congressional debate. The members who bothered to comment criticized old-age insurance for its irrelevance, pointing out that there would be a period when people would be contributing to the program and no one would be receiving regular benefits. To the members concerned about the welfare of the elderly, that hardly seemed like progress, yet they hesitated to defy Roosevelt and vote against the entire bill, including the welfare grants.

Although not a major concern of either legislative body, social insurance received considerably more scrutiny and criticism in the Senate than in the House for two important reasons. For one thing, the House had initiated action on the legislation, under the constitutional rule that tax legislation must originate there. That meant the Senate debate provided lobbyists who wished to influence the legislation with their last chance at substantive amendment. For another thing, antiadministration amendments faced a more hospitable climate in the Senate than in the House. The Senate deferred less to its standing committees than did the House and provided considerably more freedom for amendment from the floor. Further, the president exercised less control over the Senate than he did over the House. A third of the Senators, elected in 1930, had gained their seats without any help from Roosevelt and needed to worry only about the next election, when they and he would be running together.

The Senate, unlike the House, put old-age insurance to the test. Fifteen senators voted to abandon old-age insurance and remove it from the bill. Although that attempt failed, the Senate took two significant actions to weaken the bill. First, the senators, responding to pressure from the life insurance industry, removed the section dealing with the government's sale of voluntary pensions on the open market. Not surprisingly, it was the senator from Connecticut, a state with heavy insurance interests, who sponsored the amendment to delete the voluntary pensions. House conferees accepted this deletion with little protest. Second, the senators, following the lead of suggestions from private pension planners, approved an amendment that allowed private employers who already had established old-age pension plans that were as liberal as the government's Social Security plan to opt out of participating in Social Security.

Hearing of this notion, the president's advisors immediately protested. They saw this step as fatally undermining the Social Security program they had so carefully devised. If private employers could opt out of the program, they might take the best risks—young people with steady employment records—with them and leave the government to insure poorer and older people. Such a system could never be self-supporting and would ultimately collapse, discrediting the ability of the public sector to manage a large program of social benefits. The president's advisors persuaded Roosevelt of this point, and his strong pressure preserved the compulsory features of Social Security.

Neither the Senate nor the House voted a ringing endorsement of old-age insurance, and the Senate actively challenged the measure. The measure came into being because the president's predilections for social insurance coincided with those of his advisors. If anything, Roosevelt's fiscal conservatism made the plan even more cautious than his advisors recommended. The resulting Social Security program emphasized the link between contributions and benefits and hence did not pay pensions based strictly on need or chronological age. Social Security emerged not as a simple, straightforward pension law but as a very complicated piece of social machinery that few people, other than the planners and the president, wanted. On the right, people objected to the government's interference in what they considered to be the private matter of retirement. On the left, people complained about the low dollar amounts of the pensions and the fact that it would take seven years to phase the system into operation. The center held, more because of a grudging respect for the president's political power than because of conviction.

Unemployment Insurance

As Armstrong, Brown, and Latimer immersed themselves in the complicated details of old-age insurance, other members of the Committee on Economic Security staff attended to the more immediate and less tractable problem of unemployment. The staff assigned to unemployment compensation far outnumbered the staff working on old-age insurance. In general, the committee devoted more of its time

The Social Security Crisis

and attention to unemployment than to old-age security. For all of the resources devoted to the problem, however, the results proved to be less than satisfactory. If old-age insurance represented a policy innovation and an eventual landmark of the American welfare state, unemployment compensation, as the social insurance measure dealing with laid-off workers came to be called, simply channelled new legislation into existing molds.

Old-age insurance created a new federal responsibility for the security of elderly civilians, as part of a plan devised by experts in the absence of immediate partisan political pressure. Unemployment compensation, by way of contrast, bore the imprint of longstanding intellectual conflicts among the experts themselves that led in 1935 to the dismissal of federal responsibility for an important area of social policy. Bitterly divided on the best way to handle the matter, the planners failed to bring the same sense of intellectual discovery to this subject that they did to old-age security. Their stubborn pride of authorship inhibited creativity.

Ironically, between 1920 and 1935, social insurance authorities lavished more thought on the problem of unemployment compensation than on any other area of social insurance, and they produced impressive results. Madison, Wisconsin, the state capital and site of the state university, emerged as America's leading center for theoretical work related to unemployment compensation plans. By 1934, when the Committee on Economic Security began its work, Wisconsin had already gone from theory to practice and passed an unemployment compensation program. Although Wisconsin's formal jurisdiction stopped at its boundaries, its approach to social legislation influenced the entire nation and helped to set the terms for a debate over the government's response to unemployment that began in 1920, persisted through the Social Security Act's passage, and remains alive.

From the very beginning of this debate, the professors and administrators who made social insurance their specialty recognized that unemployment constituted a more sensitive risk than old-age. Few people feigned old age; most people had some proof of age, and little was expected of them, except to retire with dignity. Unemployment, to a degree that varied by circumstance, involved individual discretion. One person, laid-off from a job, scrambled to find another one or started mowing lawns or repairing toasters in his basement; another person, laid-off from the same job, decided to be unemployed. Unemployment, a nebulous term, represented a form of social invention as much as it described an objective condition, and consequently it provided a politically insecure base for social benefits. A program paying money to able-bodied people who were neither too young nor too old to work demanded the greatest caution. During a depression, that caution needed to be extreme.

Given the circumstances of the Depression, it was surprising that the Roosevelt administration attempted an unemployment compensation program at all. Unemployment compensation persisted as a subject of political inquiry in part because the Depression, although complicating the efforts of planners, made the subject a difficult one to ignore and in part because of Wisconsin's influence on the social insurance experts.

During the first three decades of the century, John R. Commons, an economics professor at the University of Wisconsin, designed social insurance programs for Wisconsin that were America's first social insurance programs. Workers' compensation, the first of these programs (enacted in 1911), greatly influenced the second, unemployment compensation (enacted in 1932). In each of these pioneering state programs, Commons differentiated his approach from earlier, European approaches to social insurance, in which the state undertook to improve the conditions of employment. In Commons's view, the employer, rather than the state, should serve as the focal point of social action. The state should regulate employment conditions in a way that prohibited unsocial behavior, but it should not become intimately involved in providing social benefits. If the employer injured his employee, he should be forced to pay for the consequences of his actions. That became the essence of the 1911 workers' compensation law. If the employer laid off an employee, he should also be required to bear some of the costs. That idea motivated the 1932 unemployment compensation law.

Commons wanted to transfer the notion of "experience rating" found in private insurance to public insurance. Private insurers tried to match the premium, or price of the insurance policy, with the risk involved. An 88-year-old diabetic paid more for life insurance than did a 24-year-old member of the Olympic track team. Buying property insurance, a pyromaniac would encounter more difficulties and higher prices than would the town fire chief. Something similar applied to both workers' compensation and unemployment compensation.

Workers' compensation covered the costs of industrial accidents. To meet these costs, state governments, such as the one in Madison, passed regulations that required employers to buy special insurance. Although the insurance requirement was mandatory, the state allowed the rates that the insurance companies charged to employers to "vary with experience," as the expression went. An employer whose factory was free of accidents paid a lower insurance premium than did a competitor whose factory was the site of many accidents that occurred on the job. The practice of differentiating rates to reflect the company's "claims experience" became known as "experience rating."

Commons applied a similar approach to the problem of unemployment when designing the state's first unemployment compensation bill in 1921. Named after the state senator who sponsored it, the Huber Bill made unemployment compensation the exclusive concern of employers and imposed a penalty on employers who laid off workers. An employer who could keep his workers employed through good times and bad would pay less than a competitor who let his people go at the first sign of economic trouble. Throughout the 1920s, the Huber Bill failed to pass, in part because representatives of the lumber industry, which regularly laid off workers during certain seasons of the year, opposed it.

The discussion sparked by the bill led to "employer reserves," a refinement of the Commons approach to unemployment insurance. Under "employer reserves," each employer paid the costs of unemployment benefits. The state, rather than an insurance company, held a company's money, but it did not mingle one employer's account with another employer's account. A company set aside money that would be used to pay a deferred wage to its laid-off worker, but not to pay for unemployment caused by some other employer. The worker gained some protection against the hardship of being unemployed; the employer received an incentive not to lay off employees, because the employer's unemployment tax rate varied with the level of his reserve fund. An employer with a full fund paid less than another employer whose fund was constantly being depleted by laid-off workers.

In 1932, Wisconsin passed the nation's first unemployment compensation law, and, a little more than two years later, Wisconsin officials, among them Edwin Witte—a Commons student, Commons's colleague in the Department of Economics, and in 1931 the head of the state's Legislative Drafting Service and hence an author of the Wisconsin law—found themselves in staff positions with the Committee on Economic Security, in charge of suggesting a federal, rather than a state, plan for unemployment compensation. It was natural that they use their own law as a model and look for a means of encouraging other states to pass similar laws.

It helped that a legislative vehicle for accomplishing this result already existed. Named after Senator Robert Wagner (D-N.Y.) and Representative David Lewis (D-Md.), the Wagner-Lewis Bill relied on an idea devised in 1933 by Justice Louis Brandeis, who discreetly passed it along to his daughter Elizabeth and her husband Paul Raushenbush, both of whom had studied with Commons and taught at the University of Wisconsin. The bill proposed the creation of a new federal payroll tax of 5 percent. If a state passed an unemployment insurance plan and the employer contributed to it, then the federal government essentially forgave the new tax. The technical term was a "tax off-set"—the contribution to the state unemployment fund "off-set" the federal tax.

Wisconsin officials, advising the Committee on Economic Security, urged the adoption of the tax off-set scheme; and their views prevailed in the committee, in the legislation that the committee prepared, and in the Social Security Act itself.

Although the Wisconsin officials successfully infused the policy process with their point of view, they encountered opposition from two sources. Part of the opposition came from owners of small businesses and others who felt that the nation could not afford an unemployment compensation program. Lloyd A. Peck, speaking on behalf of the National Association of Laundryowners, warned Congress that the new tax "will act as a definite curb on business expansion and will likely eliminate businesses now on the verge of bankruptcy." Another part of the opposition came from people who favored a federal law over a series of state laws.

Edwin Witte and his allies had three reasons for preferring state laws. First, a state system would allow the Wisconsin program to survive. Second, a state system stood a better chance of being declared constitutional by the Supreme Court. The tax off-set scheme, complicated as it was, required that each state pass an unemployment compensation law. Thus, if the federal act were declared unconstitutional, the state laws would remain. And as one academic explained, "there is no question that [the states] have the right to set up their own laws and regulate their own conditions." The third reason to prefer a state system was that it would permit states to experiment with different forms of unemployment compensation, rather than having one rigid standard set for the nation. Although Labor Secretary Perkins, for example, was not in complete sympathy with the Wisconsin approach, she did not want to "freeze the mold," but rather wished to gain experience with different forms of unemployment compensation laws. Twenty years of experimentation, she believed, would produce a "better system" than would upholding one point of view.

President Roosevelt agreed with his secretary of labor. "We've got to keep a lot of responsibility and a lot of functions in the states," he confided to Perkins; "Just think what it would be like to have all the power in the federal government if Huey Long should become President."

An odd collection of liberal reformers and cautious businessmen, who agreed on little else, opposed Perkins and favored a single, federal unemployment compensation program. Liberals, such as Paul Kellogg, the influential editor of the *Survey* magazine, wanted a federal law because they thought it would lead to more generous benefits. Kellogg advocated payroll taxes as high as five percent to fund unemployment benefits. Some businessmen, who opposed payroll taxes above three percent, nonetheless wanted the federal government to run unemployment compensation. Federal administration, they believed, would make it easier to require that employees pay part of the cost so as, in one businessman's words, "to induce a stronger sense of responsibility among employees in preventing the unemployment insurance system from being exploited by a minority." Other businessmen thought the federal government might allow them to keep existing private unemployment plans and might permit large discounts for maintaining a stable work force, and thus give them an edge over their smaller competitors.

The disparate nature of this coalition undermined its effectiveness. Disagreements over the exact design of a federal law, combined with President Roosevelt's clear preference for state laws, insured that the Committee on Economic Security would recommend a modified version of the Wagner-Lewis tax off-set scheme.

The debate over a federal plan for unemployment compensation masked a fundamental source of disagreement between the admirers and the detractors of the Commons approach to social policy. Each side accepted certain broad principles, such as the need to restrict benefits to people who had once worked and to limit the amount of time that a person could collect benefits. Unemployment benefits were not lifetime entitlements and were not supposed to be the same thing as welfare benefits or the "dole." Beyond these areas of agreement, the debate involved whether it was the employer or the government that had the ultimate responsibility for alleviating the effects of unemployment.

Commons and his followers, who might be called the Wisconsin school, wanted to make each employer responsible for his own actions. Accordingly, they favored segregating each employer's contributions and forcing each company to pay for the benefits received by its laid-off employees. It followed that they wished to restrict contributions to employers—it was, after all, not the employee's fault that he had been laid off, and if it were, then the employee should not be eligible for benefits—and to vary the rates charged. Such an arrangement preserved the role of the state as a regulator of private actions, rather than an initiator of public benefits. The state played the part of the honest cop, just making sure that the worker got what was coming to him.

In a more philosophical sense, the Wisconsin school thought of unemployment compensation as exactly that, as compensation or a form of deferred wage, similar to sick leave or a temporary retirement pension, that the company owed its employees. Unemployment compensation marked a step toward a living wage, based on an annual pay check that the employee would receive even if he were laid off for part of the year. Industry had an obligation to pay this wage and either keep its employees working throughout the year or pay them for the time lost during a layoff. But the employer had no obligation to subsidize what Eastman Kodak treasurer Marion Folsom called the "casuals, the inefficients, those who might have jobs during very good times and no jobs during bad times." Such casuals required different sorts of help from the state, such as welfare or rehabilitation.

The opponents of the Wisconsin school favored something known as "pooled funds," in which all employers put their money into one large pot. When someone became unemployed, the state, dipping into the pot, paid an unemployment benefit. Since everyone's money was mingled together, one could not tell just whose money would end up in an unemployed worker's pocket; but that mattered less to the Wisconsin opponents than did the adequacy of benefits. Hence, they advocated something akin to the English model, in which employers, employees, and the government all contributed to an unemployment fund and in which employers paid a standard rate, whatever their individual record in reducing unemployment, and employees received a standard benefit. Unemployment compensation, in this model, reflected society's obligation to the unemployed, funded by those with a stake in the community's survival, rather than a form of deferred wage payable by the employer.

Supporters of employer reserves argued the superiority of unemployment compensation, which they favored, over unemployment insurance, advocated by their opponents. The former represented benefits that an employee had earned by working; the latter guaranteed benefits to all who were not working. Pooled arrangements, in this view, amounted to a form of charity, a subsidy from efficient to inefficient employers that would encourage unemployment and result in high costs. Invoking the term for the charity campaigns of the era, one businessman called them a "new community chest of expense to all."

Opponents of employer reserves stressed the futility of applying the Wisconsin principles in an era of massive economic failure. In a time of great unemployment, they noted, it made little sense to talk of employer incentives to maintain a stable work force. All employers tried to reduce turnover and regularize employment, rather than, in one cynic's words, "sitting around waiting to get an exemption of 1 or 2 percent." With unemployment a pressing reality, the country needed to gather together as much money as possible and begin a system of unemployment insurance that paid adequate benefits; the deeper the pool of contributions, the more adequate the benefits.

Some labor leaders raised special objections to the Wisconsin approach based on their fears that it would undermine the already precarious position of unions. In their view, the employer already possessed too much control over the employee and could be expected to oppose benefits that raised labor's social wage and made it harder to lay off workers. The more control granted management, they stressed, the lower the amount of the benefits. William Green, the head of the American Federation of Labor, also worried that if contributions were segregated by employers, employers would use the money as a weapon against trade unions, perhaps by agreeing to higher reserves in return for the workers' consent not to join a union.

Searching for the right metaphors, an unsympathetic economist portrayed the Wisconsin approach as a requirement that all employers start a small bank account and the opponents' approach as forcing employers to pay premiums on one large insurance policy. He concluded that the latter approach would be "cheaper," an economist's euphemism for better and more efficient, because "the risk is spread over a much wider area."

This intellectual debate ended with an edict in favor of the Wisconsin approach rather than a creative synthesis of the two approaches. Witte, of the Committee on Economic Security staff, Perkins of the committee itself, and President Roosevelt began with a commitment to the Wagner-Lewis bill and never wavered. As a result, the political proprietors short-circuited the intellectual discovery process that had produced old-age insurance and relied instead on ideas developed as many as fifteen years earlier by Commons and his students. None of the three wanted Congress to become embroiled in potentially divisive debate over the finer points of unemployment.

Congress appreciated this point of view for four reasons. First, the congressmen tended to favor state programs over federal programs because decentralized administration offered greater patronage opportunities and more chances for local congressmen to claim credit for individual benefits. Second, they preferred to hand over politically delicate questions, such as the level of payroll taxes, to state legislatures and allow the members of those bodies to accept the inevitable criticism of business or labor organizations. Third, members of congress lacked the academicians' interests in social theory and did not wish to debate the relative merits of pooled funds and individual reserves. To them, such matters appeared to be details that could be worked out once the real decision—whether or not to start an unemployment compensation program—was made. Fourth, members brought strong regional interests to the design of social programs, and that predisposed them to remove certain policy questions, such as equal treatment of blacks, from national discussion.

Congressional impatience with the finer points of unemployment compensation also reflected the program's lack of connection with more urgent political concerns. Like old-age insurance, unemployment compensation was a program for the future. Someone who belonged to the twenty percent of the labor force already out of work might benefit immediately from the public works projects of the WPA. That program meant bread on the table. The unemployment compensation program was less relevant, because someone already out of work was, by definition, not covered by the program. Someone unemployed in August 1935 would have to wait for the state to pass an unemployment law and for the law to become effective, would have to get a new job and spend some time there, and would then have to be laid off from the new job in order for the unemployment compensation law to have any meaning whatsoever.

It was no wonder, then, that Congress handled unemployment compensation so capriciously. The House Committee on Ways and Means, without much thought or discussion, mandated that states have pooled funds. The Senate Finance Committee then simply removed the requirement and left the states on their own. In the end, as Witte told Congress, the states received, "complete freedom to establish any kind of unemployment system they wish."

In retrospect, one can see that the decision to let the states handle unemployment deserved more consideration. It was the wrong decision. On the surface, it mattered little whether an unemployed worker went to a state or federal office to pick up his check. Beneath the surface, it mattered a great deal, as the subsequent operation of the program revealed.

Consider, in this regard, how the program might function in the state of Michigan. Faced with an inquiry from an unemployed auto worker about available jobs, a state unemployment official in Lansing might consult a list and tell the unemployed worker about a job in Kalamazoo. Jobs in Houston, Texas seldom, if ever, appeared on the list, because telling workers about opportunities in Texas would violate the best interests of the state of Michigan. If the worker decided to move to Texas, he would receive money from the state of Michigan and spend it in Texas. Going to Texas, he diminished Michigan's influence over national policy by reducing the state's population and hence the size of the congressional delegation. State officers, therefore, never gained an incentive to develop a national job exchange and for that reason never did so. Meanwhile, each state used the device of experience-rating to lower unemployment taxes, in an effort to discourage employers from leaving and as a way to attract new employers.

Despite little evidence of the state governments' superiority in administering unemployment compensation, the law forces laid-off workers to go to state offices, rather than to the federal government, if they want to file a claim for unemployment compensation. The local office checks with the employer to make sure that the employee was not fired and then initiates the paperwork that leads to the worker's check. The amount of the check varies by the worker's previous wage. After a few weeks, the state office may request that a worker stop by the local employment service where, in most states, the unemployed worker states his occupation and the state officials try to match the code for the worker's occupation with the code for available job openings. No effort is made to force the worker to accept a job that does not match his stated occupation. A history professor, for example, need not accept a job as a hod carrier.

This program stands as a direct legacy of the 1935 Social Security Act, the undisputed source of social welfare policy in modern America. The judgment of economist Henry Aaron does not appear to be extreme: "When future historians review the social legislation of the first two centuries of American history," Aaron writes, "they are likely to hail the Social Security Act as the most important piece of legislation in the entire period, with the possible exception of the Homestead Act."

In 1935, Social Security loomed much less prominently as a legislative landmark. Although people recognized old-age insurance and unemployment compensation as new, even innovative, programs, they failed to see their relevance to contemporary conditions. Instead, they regarded them as the self-interested work of experts who wished to use a fortuitous political moment to advance a longstanding agenda. The substitution of orderly social insurance programs for the unruly operation of state welfare programs and federal veterans programs and the application of the social principles developed in Wisconsin stood at the top of that agenda. Despite their passion for order, however, the experts failed to predict, and hence to control, the course of future events. Social insurance developed in unexpected ways that, ultimately, led to just the sort of crisis the program planners had hoped to avoid.

3   The Triumph of Social Security, 1936–1954

Congress, which had gone along with old-age insurance but had not been happy about it, spent the next fifteen years either ignoring the program or criticizing it. Then, with little warning, Social Security became transformed into the nation's most popular social program, and politicians fell all over themselves claiming credit for its enactment and singing its praises.

As the situation stood in 1939, the economy, despite a short spurt of recovery, from the summer of 1935 until October 1937, remained depressed. The unemployment rate for 1939 reached 17.2 percent. President Franklin Roosevelt, despite a landslide victory in 1936, no longer enjoyed the enthusiastic support of an acquiescent Congress. As for the old-age insurance program, it, too, offered little in the way of economic or political encouragement. Four years after its enactment, the program had yet to pay its first regular benefits; and the legislation, as written, called for workers to have 6 percent of their salaries taken away from them by 1949 in order to receive Social Security pensions that were about half the size of pensions available at no cost from state welfare programs. "There may be some Senator who can justify that. If there is, I wish he would make a statement to the workers of the Nation," said Senator Sheridan Downey of California. Before he yielded his seat to Richard Nixon, in 1950, Downey made a career of finding fault with Social Security.

A little more than a decade after Downey spoke, circumstances changed. By 1959, with the country a generation removed from the Great Depression, the White House under Republican control, and Social Security taxes still below 6 percent, Social Security had become the largest social insurance program in the United States, and it compared favorably with private insurance. Social Security exceeded the coverage of all the private pension plans in the United States, amounted to nearly one-half of the face value of all the life insurance in the nation, and cost less than private insurance to administer. It accomplished all of these feats, in the words of one influential official, without sacrificing the American virtues of "self-responsibility."

The Politics of Social Security Finance, 1935–1939

After the passage of the Social Security Act in 1935, program administrators discovered that, despite good intentions, somehow no social welfare program could be excused from the routines of practical politics. President Roosevelt, the master politician, gave the critics of Social Security an opening through which to attack. In the president's zeal to save future generations from debt, he authorized a self-sustaining program. He proposed to gather enough money through payroll taxes to pay benefits without ever having to borrow from general revenues.

Following the president's lead, program administrators made meticulous plans for the future. At first, they expected the money coming in to greatly outstrip the money going out. In 1937, when workers discovered a Social Security deduction of 1 percent in their depleted paychecks, $511 million would arrive in the treasury, and only $6 million would be needed for administrative and other expenses. That left $505 million that the government could put in the bank and save for the day when there would be more older people in the population and when more of the older people would be eligible for Social Security. That would be the day of financial reckoning.

The government banked the money, but in a most unconventional way. The government invested its Social Security windfall in government securities or, to put it another way, in itself. In effect, the government loaned itself money and then promised to pay itself back in the future. In this way, the government acted as both the owner and the customer of the bank. Much like a private citizen, the government bought U.S. savings bonds and then, unlike a private citizen, turned around and spent the money. That meant that the Social Security money helped to finance the government's current operations, such as welfare payments, public works, or the army's payroll.

This unconventional method of banking the money figured prominently in Social Security's future. In 1967, workers would pay higher Social Security taxes, since three percent of their wages would now be withheld; but even with matching contributions from their employers it would not be enough to cover current costs. Congress would have to dip into the bank account, called the "reserve," and use some of the money that had accumulated to pay the benefits. By 1980, planners expected the money in the special Social Security bank to reach more than $46 billion.

From the vantage point of 1937, when payroll deductions began, the Social Security financing scheme possessed the fantastic qualities of science fiction. In the first place, $46 billion constituted an enormous amount of money, about eight times the amount of money then in circulation. In the second place, the scheme forced the government to behave in a manner that strained credulity. It required federal authorities simply to allow the money to pile up in the special bank, ignoring incessant pleas to spend the money on one worthy project or another.

The elderly possessed a special claim to the hypothetical money in this paper bank. To serve the cause of prudent management, the president expected the elderly to wait for five years before they received social security benefits. Between 1937 and 1942, workers and their employers would pay Social Security taxes, even though no one would receive regular benefits in those years. As older people lingered in the far-from-hospitable labor force, struggling to find any available jobs, the money continued to pile up—at least in theory—in the treasury's special social security bank.

With plans to collect so much money and give it to so few people, the Social Security program became a natural target of the president's political rivals. "Such a treasure—all in one place and conveniently eligible for Congressional raids throughout the years—is an utterly naive conception," argued Michigan's Republican senator Arthur Vandenberg. "That it would remain intact and not suffer periodical depletions is more than human nature in a political democracy can rationally anticipate." Alfred Landon, the 1936 Republican candidate for president, described Social Security as "unjust, unworkable, stupidly drafted and wastefully financed."

Landon, Vandenberg, and other opponents of Social Security reasoned that the president had outsmarted himself. Surpluses, although necessary to keep future tax rates within reasonable limits and to forestall the use of general revenues, created the very problems that they were intended to avoid. Surpluses encouraged politicians to make the program more liberal, just as large surpluses in the late-nineteenth-century federal budget had been used as a justification for expanding veterans' programs. A liberalized program would defeat all the efforts at planning for the future. When the time came to reach into the bank account, there would be no money on hand because the surplus would already have been spent. Landon and Vandenberg believed that the program that had so carefully planned its financial future would crash in a mountain of debt. It would exemplify bad social planning, just as the Townsend plan had.

In his futile effort to avoid future difficulties, the president also created serious immediate problems. Social Security taxes reduced the size of many workers' paychecks and in so doing deprived the economy of money that could have been spent on groceries, clothes, cars, or houses. At best, the Social Security tax did no harm because it took money from workers and gave it to the government, which spent it on the salaries of government workers and government contractors. At worst, the tax depleted the money supply, depressed demand, and reduced prices. At a time of deflation and shrinking investment, argued the English economist John Maynard Keynes in a 1936 book that would influence economic theory for the next forty years, the government should pump money into the economy, not suck it out through rising taxes.

Tensions heightened when the first Social Security deductions began to show up in workers' paychecks in January 1937. Social Security, just started and already discredited, faced major challenges by workers, businessmen, and the states. Workers wondered just where their money was going; employers resented the paperwork involved in computing the deductions. Workers objected to the reduction in their take-home pay; employers protested new taxes that cut into their profits. Soon, the economy began to weaken; and some people, in honor of the Social Security deductions, named the dangerous downturn the "Social Security recession." The states, for their part, viewed Social Security as a threat to their political systems and to their autonomy.

Beyond all of these threats to the program's survival lay the haunting fear that the Supreme Court would rule the legislation unconstitutional and invalidate it. Many of the New Deal programs that passed in 1933 failed to survive the Court's scrutiny. Roosevelt hoped to spare the 1935 programs, including the Social Security Act, a similar fate—if necessary by packing the Court with sympathetic judges. On February 5, 1937, he sent Congress a plan that gave him the power to appoint as many as six new justices to the Supreme Court. In a famous outburst, Hatton Sumners, the chairman of the House Judiciary Committee, said, "Boys, here's where I cash in my chips."

As the president presented his controversial plan to reorganize the federal courts, the Supreme Court pondered the constitutionality of the old-age insurance and unemployment compensation programs. The test case for old-age insurance involved a shareholder in the Edison Electric Illuminating Company of Boston who argued that the deductions from employees' paychecks produced "unrest" and demands for increased wages, even as the company suffered "irreparable loss" because of deteriorating business conditions. The company's lawyers spoke of how paternal government aid sapped the "virtues of self-reliance and frugality" and bred "a race of weaklings." The government, represented by Robert Jackson and Charles Wyzanski, who later became prominent federal judges, countered that the Social Security Act simply exercised the federal government's constitutional power to tax.

On May 24, 1937, Justice Cardozo announced the Court's opinion to a full chamber. The audience eagerly waited to see if the trend begun the month before would continue. The previous spring, the Court had found a New York State minimum wage law unconstitutional. Then, in March 1937, Justice Owen Roberts reversed his position, and the Court decided, by a one-vote margin, to uphold a Washington State minimum wage statute similar to the New York law it had overturned only a year before. Two weeks later, Roberts stayed with the majority as the Court ruled in favor of the Wagner Act establishing the right of workers to bargain collectively with management through representatives of their own choosing. Now came the Social Security decision.

Cardozo, in an eloquently worded decision, continued to take the Court along the New Deal path. In two 5-4 decisions, the Court validated the unemployment insurance provisions of the Social Security Act and, in a third decision, upheld the constitutionality of old-age insurance by a 7-2 margin. In the words of one young federal bureaucrat who attended the oral arguments and returned to the Court to hear the decision, Cardozo delivered his opinions with a "cadence and power of language indicating his sense of their historic and far-reaching significance." "The hope behind this statute," the Justice said, in words that were to find their way into a generation of textbooks, "is to save men and women from the rigors of the poorhouse as well as from the haunting fear that such a lot awaits them when journey's end is near."

Even as the Court affirmed the federal government's role in old-age security, the states, of necessity, remained the major providers of old-age pensions. With the federal government still mired in its prudent planning stage, gathering money that would be paid in 1942 to citizens who were not yet old in 1937, the state authorities faced the delicate and demanding task of deciding just which of the needy elderly would receive immediate aid. Conflict between federal administrators, responsible for overseeing federal grants to the states for old-age pensions, and state authorities, responsible for administering the grants, soon arose.

On one level, the dispute involved differing visions of social policy. The federal administrators regarded themselves as professionals in the business of substituting national social insurance for local welfare. They viewed their major objectives, as they established 42.6 million Social Security accounts and handled 3,000 daily requests for information, as removing politics from public programs and demonstrating that the public sector could deliver benefits with businesslike efficiency. They defined the removal of politics to mean that pensions would be awarded on the basis of income and family condition, rather than political preference or location. Efficiency implied quantifiable measures of competence, such as answering letters within 72 hours. Many of the state and local administrators still viewed themselves as politicians in charge of dispensing local patronage, rather than as social welfare professionals. Showing little interest in replacing a local welfare system with a remote, nationally oriented program of social insurance, they wanted to spend the federal grants for old-age pensions on their own terms and fought hard to preserve the local welfare system. In so doing, they reduced the level of support for an already badly beleaguered old-age insurance program.

Not surprisingly, then, the federal administrators hesitated to give money to the local officials without reassurances that the money would be awarded according to the rules that the federal bureaucrats had devised. Neither side wished to follow the dictates of the other.

On another level, the dispute concerned parochial politics of the sort that divided President Roosevelt and the national Democratic party from local politicians. The president, like the local politicians, wanted to reward his friends. Events in Ohio between 1935 and 1940 revealed both levels of the dispute.

In 1934, Martin L. Davey, a businessman who was hostile to the social programs of the New Deal, beat a candidate sympathetic to President Roosevelt in the Democratic primary. In 1935 Davey became the governor, fired the previous director of state relief, suspended civil service regulations that required county welfare directors to have social work degrees, and engaged in a pitched battle with Harry Hopkins, the federal relief administrator, at one point swearing out a warrant for Hopkins's arrest. When it came time to release federal funds for old-age pensions in Ohio, administrators proved less than eager. According to the federal officials, Governor Davey used the state's old-age pension rolls as a way of insuring political loyalty. Elderly pensioners, many of whom exercised their right to vote, received constant reminders that they owed their payments to the beneficence of Governor Davey. Just before one Christmas, for example, they learned that a 10 percent increase in their benefits had been ordered by the governor.

Federal officials decided to test their power against the state and intervene. Right before the 1938 gubernatorial primary, Davey wrote to all old-age assistance recipients, reminding them of how he had raised their benefits and requesting that they talk to their friends and relatives and "ask them to go to the polls without fail on primary election day . . . and ask for a Democratic ballot, in order to vote for me." Arthur Altmeyer, the chairman of the Social Security Board, denounced Davey's action and ordered an inquiry into Ohio's welfare practices to determine if the state was complying with the law. Davey, who refused to cooperate with the inquiry, lost the primary. Altmeyer released a report that condemned Ohio's practice of raising pension levels without regard to individual need, the state's accounting procedures, and its means of handling complaints. The federal government refused to reimburse the state for its October 1938 welfare expenditures and ultimately withheld more than a million dollars from Ohio. In November the Democrats lost the state's gubernatorial election.

Arthur Altmeyer saw the Ohio incident as part of a national pattern in which "the old age assistance laws were used by candidates for office and the recipients were deluged with campaign literature and promises, counterpromises, and warnings and counterwarnings and that created a very bad situation." He agreed with New York City's Commissioner of Welfare, who worked for Fiorello LaGuardia, the city's fiercely independent mayor, that the nation had a choice. According to the New York commissioner, welfare programs could be administered "economically, efficiently, and humanely" or they could be "operated on the basis of political patronage." Competent people, defined as those with "education, training, and experience" could administer the programs or government could "turn the whole matter over to the political machines and ruin the Nation's programs for the aid of persons in need of governmental assistance."

Despite the influence their inquiry had on the 1938 governor's election in Ohio, the federal administrators regarded their actions in Ohio as a warning that they would punish states that mixed old-age assistance and politics, not as a political move of their own. They believed that, because the Social Security Board was bipartisan and demonstrated "a special knowledge of the law and its operations," it possessed a competence that elevated it above conventional political institutions such as Congress and the courts. Governor Davey accused the federal officials of "insulting tactics" and "dirty politics."

Incensed by the federal decision to withhold funds from the state, members of Ohio's congressional delegation chose to use Congress as a means of getting the money back. They persuaded their colleagues to pass a law in 1940 that restored the funds. Arthur Altmeyer, not to be outdone, prevailed on President Roosevelt to veto the law. This action further enraged those sympathetic to Ohio's plight, who railed that "one little bureaucrat appointed to his office because he may have written a magazine article" proved "more powerful than a Congress and a Senate elected by the people." Still, the congressmen did not have the votes to override the veto, the measure failed, and the appointed experts scored a victory over the politicians.

This victory, like the Supreme Court's approval, mattered little if the Social Security program failed to take hold as a major social program. In 1938, an endorsement from the Townsendites still meant more votes in a local election than did defending Social Security. One Ohio politician maintained that the Townsend movement held the balance of power in many sections of that state.

Although the professionals who administered Social Security fancied themselves to be above politics, they gradually realized that no system of social benefits could exist in a political vacuum but instead required a solid base of political support. By the end of the 1930s, the president could no longer shield Social Security from harsh congressional criticism; and Arthur Altmeyer, among others, began to see the necessity of actively fighting for old-age insurance's political survival. As early as October 1937, he started to think of ways to recast Social Security in a socially responsible but politically palatable way. He realized that the reserve method of financing was a liability and should be jettisoned. What began as an effort to rise above politics by budgeting for the future and revealing the system's ultimate costs ended up mired in politics.

Altmeyer now wanted Congress to abandon the reserve system by liberalizing benefits and beginning the payment of benefits sooner than the scheduled starting date of 1942. He hoped to accomplish these results and still preserve the features of social insurance in which benefits were related to contributions and in which care was taken to keep costs within manageable limits. To work out the complicated logistics, Senator Vandenberg and Altmeyer agreed to form a special advisory council that met throughout 1938 and formulated the changes in Social Security that became law in 1939.

In the new atmosphere of the late 1930s, the public image of the Social Security program changed considerably, as part of the self-conscious campaign to make the program more politically appealing. Social Security's defenders now sought to sharpen the distinctions between social insurance and welfare and to explain how social insurance better served America's needs in a world beset by threats to the nation's security. In 1935, Douglas Brown and his colleagues had defended the old-age insurance program as something already established and tested in Europe and as a responsible way of meeting future expenditures that would, in effect, *complement* welfare. In 1939, Douglas Brown and Arthur Altmeyer defended old-age insurance as an *alternative* to welfare and as a distinctively American program that would protect this country from the evils that had befallen Europe.

Brown, in a masterful appearance before Congress in 1939, elegantly formulated the new defense of Social Security. He criticized welfare, noting that it involved "mounting dependency and the impairment of independence and incentive." Nor did the harm end there. Relief in the form of welfare led to "paternalism," the state treating the citizen as a child. The more helpless the citizen became, the more relief he would receive. And once the state gained that sort of power, it became an agent of corruption and destruction. If Americans wanted graphic evidence of this tendency, they had only to look at Hitler's Germany and Stalin's Russia, where the state reigned supreme and suppressed individuality. Brown concluded that America should not fall into the trap of welfare and should opt for social insurance instead. Old-age insurance prevented dependency, because it emphasized "thrift and self-reliance." As a consequence, old-age insurance maintained the "dignity of human personality," which was "certainly needed in these days of totalitarianism."

Such rhetoric, although politically prudent, nonetheless ignored many features of Social Security. In social insurance, low-wage and short-term earners received more for their money because administrative authorities assumed that their needs were greater. As in a welfare program, Social Security substituted the judgment of a group of bureaucrats, acting in the name of the state, for what Brown had called "thrift and self-reliance." Furthermore, both Brown and Altmeyer, contrary to their political rhetoric, wanted to move Social Security further in the direction of paternalism.

Family benefits, as proposed by federal administrators in 1938 and adopted by Congress in 1939, became the chosen vehicle. Describing the major changes made in 1939, Arthur Altmeyer spoke of a "family concept." The essence of this concept involved four features of the Social Security amendments of 1939. First, the amendments established new benefits for elderly retirees and widows; second, they created new benefits for the survivors of workers who died before retirement age; third, they changed the way in which all benefits were computed; fourth, they provided that the elderly would not have to wait until 1942 to receive benefits and that, instead, benefits would begin almost immediately.

Each of the four features, by increasing the amount of paternalism in the Social Security program, heightened the similarities between Social Security and welfare, just at the time when program defenders began to emphasize the differences. In welfare, the state, by taking care of its needy citizens, acted as a father would toward his children. In the post-1939 Social Security program, should a working father die, the state would start payments to the mother and the other surviving family members. In so doing, the state acted as the father's replacement and, in effect, assumed his role as the breadwinner. To start a program of family protection, the state necessarily acted in a paternalistic manner by making decisions concerning how a family should function, decisions that, as in the welfare program, had nothing to do with Brown's notions of "thrift and self-reliance."

New benefits for the elderly also reflected paternalistic social judgments that had nothing to do with a worker's Social Security contributions. Married couples would now get more than single people. A retired bachelor received a full benefit that was actually slightly less than he would have received under the original law, but a married couple acquired a full benefit for the husband and an additional half benefit for the wife. On average, married couples would collect 150 percent of what bachelors received, even if a single worker and a married worker put exactly the same amount into the fund. "I don't mind taxing the bachelors. I think they ought to take on the responsibility of sharing their income with someone else," a member of the 1938 advisory council said.

As an example of the subtle calculations involved, consider the case of a single man and a married man, both of whom worked for 35 years at an average wage of $50 a month. Under the 1935 plan, both workers would have earned a benefit of $30, but under one version of the 1939 plan, the single man would receive $27.50 a month, the married man $41.25.

A different sort of paternalistic reasoning applied to widows. A woman whose husband died would, if she reached the age of 65 without getting remarried, obtain a benefit equal to three-quarters of her deceased husband's full benefit. The widow, in the words of another advisory council member, needed less than a man, because "she is used to doing her own housework whereas the single man has to go to a restaurant."

Other new benefits reflected similar sorts of social judgments. These included survivors' benefits, such as the payment of a widow's benefit to a woman caring for a child under 18 and the payment of an additional benefit of 50 percent for a dependent child. The amendments also allowed for a parent's benefit, if the parent had been dependent on a deceased worker *and* if the worker had no surviving widow or child.

As was customary, the new formula for computing benefits, another feature of the 1939 law, related benefits to contributions, yet it also contained a bonus for poorer workers. For example, a worker with an average wage of $50 a month might receive a benefit of $20 a month; a worker with an average wage of $100 "earned" a benefit of $25. The higher your wage, the higher your benefit, but if your wage were twice that of another person, it did not mean that your benefit would be twice as high.

Congress accepted all of this with its usual impatience. Higher benefits always made good politics. Paying benefits sooner was always better than paying benefits later. The Democrats, furthermore, wanted to take the Social Security issue away from the Republicans by eliminating the negative talk about the huge Social Security reserve. The proposals accomplished this objective in a politically attractive manner. By raising benefit levels, they reduced the size of the hypothetical reserve. Taking money out of the bank today, they lowered the account's future balance.

At the same time, the 1939 amendments begged a question that, in retrospect, was the most important question. How would the new benefits be financed? Arthur Altmeyer hoped Congress would relinquish the reserves "with its eyes open, recognizing the future consequences of so doing." Altmeyer wished to raise the Social Security tax rate in 1940 from 2 to 3 percent of payroll, not so much for economic as for psychological reasons. He worried that if benefits were increased and tax increases postponed, the public would get the impression that, "after all, there isn't much relationship between contributions and benefits." As for the longer term, Altmeyer favored introducing general revenues into the program and splitting the cost burden evenly among employers, employees, and general revenues. He also wanted Congress to make a definite statement on how the system's future liabilities would be handled.

The members of Congress cared little about future liabilities and made no provisions for them; they saw the chance to raise benefits and reduce taxes, and they took it. The House Committee on Ways and Means gloated that by freezing the payroll tax rate at its 2 percent level, instead of raising it to 3 percent as previously planned, taxpayers would save $825 million in three years. The Committee also noted that contributory insurance served as a "safeguard against excessive liberalization of benefits," even as it proudly announced the plans for new benefits to cover aged wives, widows, and children.

As always, congressional debate centered on welfare, rather than social insurance. Members demanded that the federal government put up more of the money for state old-age pensions. In the House of Representatives, for example, a proposal appeared for a four to one federal match, up to twenty federal dollars. That meant if the state contributed five dollars, the federal government would supply twenty dollars for a total of twenty-five. The Senate concentrated on an amendment allowing a two-for-one match, up to 15 federal dollars, and on a plan for a flat grant of $40 to those in need. None of these changes became law, although several came close, and, taken together, they consumed far more legislative time than did the rest of the 1939 amendments.

Despite the changes made in 1939, old-age insurance had yet to pay benefits on a regular basis, and the benefits that it would begin to pay in 1940 would still be smaller than most welfare grants. Social Security remained small, inconsequential, and vulnerable to attack.

Wars at Home and Abroad

World War II, a foreign event that transformed domestic politics, began within a few weeks of the passage of the Social Security amendments of 1939. In time, Germany's invasion of Poland brought America's entry into the war, the end of the Depression, and major changes in social welfare policy. The war provided another reason to postpone consideration of Social Security's long-term liabilities, since an improved economy generated an impressive windfall in Social Security revenues. Beyond its effects on any one program, the war caused a major reconsideration of New Deal social policy and strengthened localities, with their traditional welfare systems, at the expense of the federal government.

The war ended the New Deal and ushered in a period of conservative social policy in America; yet other countries, notably Great Britain, reacted to their wartime experiences differently. Simply put, the war expanded the welfare state in Europe and contracted it in America, despite the strong desire on the part of social welfare administrators, such as Arthur Altmeyer, that America follow Britain's example. Altmeyer yearned for America to react as enthusiastically to proposals to expand Social Security as Britain did to the suggestions contained in what came to be known as the Beveridge report.

On November 20, 1942, Sir William Beveridge published a report entitled "Social Insurance and Allied Services." The report criticized the lack of bureaucratic coordination in British social policy and called for a national, contributory, social insurance system that would cover such contingencies as ill health, unemployment, permanent disability, old-age, and need for medical care. A worker, his employer, and the government would all make contributions and the worker would receive what authorities on both sides of the Atlantic referred to as "cradle-to-grave protection."

In 1943, American Social Security administrators formally proposed a plan that faintly echoed the Beveridge plan. Resting on the notion of coordination of social insurance at the federal level, the plan called for a system of contributory social insurance that included unemployment compensation, temporary and permanent disability payments, old-age insurance, and health insurance. The plan, in other words, would fund each of these things in the same way as old-age insurance was already funded. Workers and employers would contribute through payroll taxes collected by the federal government. In return, the federal government would provide them with a wide range of benefits.

If passed, the proposal would become our version of cradle-to-grave insurance—our welfare state—different from the Beveridge plan only in detail. Although both plans called for centralized control and highlighted social insurance, our plan placed less emphasis on governmental contributions. Instead, we insisted on benefits that reflected a worker's contributions. Beveridge stressed uniformity: all workers paid the same amount and received the same level of benefits. Our Social Security plan, to use historian Jerry Cates's phrase, "insured inequality," by varying both the contributions and the benefits to reflect a worker's income. Within important limits, richer workers paid more and received more.

The British responded far more fervently to Beveridge's ideas and rhetoric than the Americans did to this country's welfare state proposals. The British lionized Beveridge and made him a celebrity. The government sold over half a million copies of the report, and as his biographer notes, "pictures of Beveridge, looking prophetically white-haired and benign, were flashed by Pathe News into every cinema in the country."

The British moved in Beveridge's direction after the war, and the Americans veered away from the centralized, coordinated welfare state he and his American counterparts advocated. Beveridge called the war "a revolutionary moment in the world's history," which was sure to abolish "landmarks of every kind" and create a "free field." Wartime sacrifice required that the government be "ready in time with plans for [a] better world." Since we did not regard the war as

---

the same sort of landmark as did the British, it was not as important for us to build an alternative to the warfare state as it was for the British. No bombs dropped on New York as they did on London, and, although the war demanded considerable sacrifice by America, it brought considerable profit as well. For us, the war did not produce a revolution in social relations so much as it restored the prosperity to which we had become accustomed. The American government, unlike the British, owed its citizens nothing more than continuing prosperity; the private market, charity, state and local government, and voluntary associations would take care of the rest. Great Britain created a national health service, to cite just one example; the American Social Security proposal, known as the Wagner-Murray-Dingell bill, never came close to passage.

Far from solidifying the legislative accomplishments of the New Deal, the war provided an opportunity to step back and reconsider them. Some, such as the public works programs, created on an emergency basis for the Depression, easily gave way to war mobilization. People no longer needed to work paving streets or building post offices for the WPA; private employers now begged them to make jeeps and assemble fighter bombers. Other New Deal social programs, such as the welfare provisions in the Social Security Act, already allowed significant room for local discretion and authority. Wartime conditions nurtured alternatives to the New Deal programs, such as private social security plans, which were greatly expanded during and after the war.

The fate of unemployment compensation between 1935 and 1960 illustrated a more general trend in social policy away from central control and toward local responsibility.

The Social Security Act of 1935 permitted the states almost total control over their unemployment compensation plans. After the passage of the act, all of the states passed unemployment compensation laws; and, as expected, each of the states offered employers discounts on unemployment compensation, a practice similar to reducing safe drivers' automobile insurance premiums.

The subsequent development of unemployment compensation reflected wartime and postwar prosperity. Five million people drew unemployment benefits in the year before our entry into the war. In 1944, a war year, only half a million people received benefits, and after the war, when major problems were expected, Congress permitted returning veterans to receive "readjustment allowances," taking the pressure off the state systems. When the Depression ended, therefore, the states found themselves with more funds on hand than they had expected, and they proceeded to offer discounts to employers. These actions fed on themselves. If one state discounted its rates, then a neighboring state often followed because the alternative was to lose the competitive edge, to weaken the business climate. By the end of 1946, for example, forty-five states provided for experience rating, and all of the states offered it by 1947.

Discounts and low unemployment rates combined to reduce unemployment compensation taxes on employers. The Social Security Act had called for a 3 percent tax on employers' payrolls, with .3 percent retained by the federal government to fund the administration of the program and the remaining 2.7 percent returned to the states to pay benefits. By 1946, the actual tax had fallen to an average of 1.4 percent. One state attained a rate of 0.3 percent; no state charged more than 2.1 percent.

In the postwar era, with Franklin Roosevelt dead and the circumstances that produced the Social Security Act fading from memory, such practices no longer attracted much criticism. Experts, who once insisted that the federal government run the unemployment program because it would be too costly for the states to do so, now praised state administration. They portrayed the states' ability to offer discounts through experience rating as nothing less than a triumph for the American way of life. In defense of state administration, proponents of experience rating used language similar to that of Social Security's defenders. Both sets of policy analysts claimed to favor a uniquely American approach to social policy that differed from dangerous European practices. America faced a choice, as Paul Raushenbush, the head of Wisconsin's unemployment compensation program, put it, between "a centralized system of political and economic control . . . and that which experience rating seeks to promote and encourage." The European dictators, recently defeated in the war, took the centralized route. Experience rating enlisted the "brains of hundreds of thousands of American employers, managers, businessmen, and all kinds of other folk—in the common cause of improving our actual performance, under our present economic system."

Few saw the need to federalize the state unemployment programs; yet, for all of the praise, unemployment compensation also engendered a subtle backlash. From the left, federal administrators criticized the differences in the program from state to state. In 1959, for example, Alaska, Delaware, Michigan, and Pennsylvania needed to borrow money from the federal government to make unemployment payments; other states ran large surpluses.

From the right, employers surrendered their low tax rates only very reluctantly, and they encouraged close surveillance of unemployment applications to keep cheaters from the rolls and keep costs down. But this type of close monitoring defeated the original notion of unemployment benefits as a deferred wage, available as a matter of right. Popular publications added legitimacy to the search for abuse in the system. In 1960, the *Reader's Digest* reported the story of Mrs. Sheila Shaw, who drew 9 weeks of unemployment compensation after she quit her $45-a-week clerk-typist job to get married. Her employer appealed and lost.

The history of the unemployment compensation system showed that decisions made casually by Congress in 1935 produced important consequences. Created as a permissive state system, unemployment compensation never escaped its original mold. In theory, freedom to experiment meant that the states, learning from one another, sorted good practices from bad and produced the very best system. Labor Secretary Frances Perkins had subscribed to that theory in 1935. In reality, freedom to experiment became a license to lower unemployment compensation tax rates and to limit benefits. Nonetheless, federal officials never persuaded Congress to change the system, and America's approach to unemployment compensation continued to rely on state-run programs throughout the war and postwar eras.

Private social security, achieved through collective bargaining, marked another wartime legacy that put a brake on expanding the American welfare state to include cradle-to-grave protection.

The war brought both higher tax rates and higher profits to corporations and increased corporate interest in tax shelters. During the war, also, employees in mass production industries, such as automobiles and steel, were unionized, as a result of the New Deal's encouragement of organized labor. At the same time, the government attempted to control wage increases as a means of preventing inflation. Pensions and other fringe benefits therefore met the needs of employees because they were a legitimate object of collective bargaining and a disguised but legal form of pay increase. They earned the employer's approval because they helped to reduce turnover and because employer contributions could be deducted from taxable income. As a result of these forces, 2.25 million workers gained private pension coverage between 1940 and 1945, and the trend continued in the postwar era.

Asked in 1949 why trade unions put so much emphasis on private health and welfare funds, James A. Brownlee, an official of the American Federation of Labor, said, the answer was "quite simple. Because the social security law has not been amended. Because its provisions are so antiquated and unjust." Brownlee agreed with Philip Murray, of the Congress of Industrial Organizations, who asserted, "the poorer the laws, the greater emphasis we will have to put on collective bargaining supplements." Both Brownlee and Murray tended to see private and public benefits as complementing one another. "We are not afraid that Congress will do too much," said Murray, "rather we fear it will do too little."

Unless the Social Security system became more effective, Arthur Altmeyer said, there would be "demands for flat pensions, for veterans pensions, for health and welfare funds." These demands would further undermine a system that Altmeyer regarded as already seriously weakened by a lack of central direction.

In this regard, Altmeyer had traveled a long way. Once, as executive secretary of the Wisconsin Industrial Commission, he helped to implement Wisconsin's 1932 unemployment compensation law and defended its emphasis on experience rating and state administration. He hired Paul Raushenbush to administer the law and relied on Raushenbush and his wife Elizabeth Brandeis for advice. Within ten years of Altmeyer's arrival in Washington, the Raushenbushes and Altmeyers were barely speaking to one another. Altmeyer, as a federal bureaucrat, saw the advantages of federal administration through such plans as the Wagner-Murray-Dingell bill and its promise of cradle-to-grave insurance. Such a scheme promised to end the disturbing disparities in social benefits that separated Mississippi from Wisconsin, Alabama from Massachusetts. Such a scheme held the potential to replace inefficient administrators in Ohio with specially trained, more competent, and better motivated bureaucrats in Washington, D.C. It therefore disturbed Altmeyer that, even in the face of a national effort to fight the war and win the peace, much of America's social welfare system remained completely decentralized.

At home, in Madison, Raushenbush and Brandeis kept the faith, giving wartime speeches that emphasized "preserving back-home democracy in as many fields as practicable" and urging that the nation not be "stampeded by the war emergency into distortion or nationalization of a program [unemployment compensation] that might serve us well for decades to come." In the war and postwar eras, the Raushenbushes got far the better of the argument; their healthy skepticism toward a massive federal bureaucracy found more favor than did Altmeyer's vision of an efficient, centrally administered welfare state.

The Race between Welfare and Social Insurance

If Altmeyer lost the battle to control the unemployment compensation program from Washington, he nonetheless won a major expansion of old-age and survivors' insurance in 1950 that, within months, made Social Security America's largest and most important social welfare program. In this regard, Social Security represented the great exception to social policy trends of the postwar era. At a time of limited success for federal initiatives in such fields as unemployment, disability, and health care, Social Security, defined as old-age and survivors' insurance, enjoyed its greatest triumph. The 1950 Social Security amendments provided the breakthrough that brought Social Security to parity with welfare and enabled the elderly, at least, to live in a Beveridge-style welfare state. The fact that the prospects for the expansion of Social Security looked far from promising in the late 1940s made the breakthrough all the more remarkable. At the time, Social Security advocates often described Social Security politics as a race between welfare and social insurance, one that welfare was winning.

By the end of the 1940s, the numbers told a story in which welfare was much more important than social insurance. Twice as many people received welfare as received social insurance, even though America had never been richer and even though Congress had expanded social insurance in 1939. The nation spent more than three times as much on welfare as on social insurance. During the 1940s, furthermore, the level of welfare payments increased, in part because of federal legislation that increased the federal share of payments. Old-age insurance, in contrast, remained unchanged after 1939.

A closer look at the figures, however, demonstrated that welfare's importance varied by location, a fact of great political significance. Nationwide, about one out of four people over age 65 received welfare. In Louisiana, however, the rate rose to more than three out of every four elderly persons, and in New Jersey, where twice as many people received Social Security as received welfare, the rate fell to one out of ten. In Louisiana, 113,000 people received an average of $47 a month from old-age assistance (welfare), and 23,000 received an average of $16 from old-age insurance.

The key demographic factor turned out to be that rural, agricultural areas contained practically no Social Security beneficiaries. Most Social Security recipients were clustered in urban areas. Chicago, for example, housed more Social Security than welfare beneficiaries in 1948, but in the farming areas of downstate Illinois, there were twice as many people on welfare as on social insurance. Four times as many welfare recipients as Social Security recipients lived in the states of North Carolina, South Carolina, Mississippi, Tennessee, Alabama, and Georgia. And in the fourth congressional district of Texas, where the ratio of expenditures between welfare and social insurance was on the order of 36 to 1, the local congressman could honestly say, "old-age and survivors' insurance means practically nothing to us."

A similar pattern applied to the amount of welfare benefits as to the distribution of Social Security beneficiaries. The areas with more Social Security recipients tended to be places with high welfare benefits. The pattern applied both within and among states. In Indiana, one of twenty states that permitted county variations in welfare benefits, the counties in the south of the state, near the Ohio River, paid average grants of about $27.50. The northern counties, heavily industrialized and located near Chicago, managed average welfare grants of about $37.50. At the same time, December 1948, the national average monthly welfare payment to an elderly individual stood at $42. Mississippi averaged under $25; California's average payment exceeded $60.

Hoping somehow to exploit this confusing pattern, the defenders of Social Security continued to promote social insurance over welfare. In 1949, Douglas Brown pleaded with Congress to rescue Social Security, noting that although "relief" was more popular and easier to administer, unless it was promptly replaced by social insurance, it would lead the United States "down the primrose path of state paternalism." Brown compared the situation to a fairy tale with an unhappy ending. Unless Congress strengthened and enlarged social insurance, "it may become a Cinderella displaced by its more demanding step-sisters, assistance and relief." Since public assistance was "fast winning the race," it looked as though Cinderella might never go the ball.

Once again, the Social Security program faced a fundamental problem and, once again, its critics and supporters collaborated on the creation of a special advisory council to work on a compromise. The second advisory council held its first meeting in December 1947 and issued a series of reports in 1948. These reports formed the basis of the 1950 amendments to the program, just as, a decade earlier, an advisory council had laid the foundation for the 1939 amendments.

Where the 1937–38 advisory council had taken reserve financing as its major problem, the second advisory council concentrated on the race between welfare and social insurance. The council's report, a seminal document in America's social welfare history, stated its objectives quite directly as "to prevent dependency through social insurance and thus greatly reduce the need for assistance."

The council seized upon the geographic and demographic patterns that differentiated recipients of welfare and of social insurance. Its report explicitly recognized that the agricultural states were the ones with the highest disparities between welfare and social insurance, and it treated these disparities as a problem in public finance. Because employers and employees paid for social insurance but welfare came partly out of a state or county's general revenues, poorer agricultural states faced greater financial burdens in aiding the elderly than did richer industrial states. The result was that the agricultural states paid lower, less adequate benefits to a greater share of the elderly population than did the industrial states.

The statement of the problem implied a solution—the very solution that Brown, Altmeyer, and their allies had urged for over a decade—and that was to expand Social Security coverage to include rural residents and to raise Social Security benefits so that they compared favorably with welfare benefits. In other words, bring the self-employed and agricultural workers into the Social Security system and pay them benefits that would be as high as welfare benefits. The fact that rural areas paid relatively low welfare benefits eased the problem somewhat, yet the task nonetheless appeared daunting. Efforts to expand Social Security met continuing resistance from politicians who preferred to raise the federal contribution toward locally administered old-age pensions.

The advisory council decided that Social Security needed a completely "new start" to break the impasse, even though two previous starts had failed to stop the advance of welfare. First there had been the 1935 law, with its self-financing features; next, the 1939 law, with its family benefits and new benefit formula, had appeared. The advisory council hoped to launch a third start, in which benefits were raised to compete with welfare.

The council's proposal contained two basic elements. The first element involved bringing new groups into Social Security and keeping them there. That meant extending Social Security coverage and making sure that elderly individuals in these groups qualified quickly for benefits. The second element consisted of boosting benefits for everyone, to make Social Security more financially attractive than welfare.

In proposing to extend coverage, the council concentrated on regularly employed farm and domestic workers and on self-employed people not working on farms. The council hoped to bring the family maid, a regular worker on a large midwestern wheat farm, and a proprietor of the local haberdashery store into the system. Willfully ignoring previous political battles, it portrayed the barriers to participation by these groups as administrative rather than political—an inability to collect money from them. The now longer reach of the income tax lessened the difficulties. Since so many people now paid income tax, federal tax returns could be used to compute Social Security payments.

Keeping the maid, the agricultural employee, and the local businessman in the system meant making sure they qualified for higher Social Security than welfare benefits. People consumed social welfare benefits as rationally as any other product; retired people sought to maximize their incomes every bit as much as working people. Just raising the basic Social Security benefits required nothing more than legislative fiat; but more subtle problems, of the sort that had plagued Brown, Latimer, and Armstrong in 1934, remained to be solved.

These problems concerned the rules under which a person qualified for Social Security. For someone already retired from domestic or agricultural service, new benefits, even large and substantial benefits, meant little or nothing, since the only way for a retired person to get them was to stop retiring and start working. For all practical purposes, the new benefits, to paraphrase economist John Maynard Keynes, could as well have been on the moon. Once again, the rule that required a person to "pay before he could play" created difficulties that impeded Social Security's progress.

The council decided to bend the rule as much as it could without contorting it beyond recognition. In the council's recommendation, one still needed to pay to play and those already retired, having never paid, could never receive a Social Security benefit; however, the council decided to offer workers nearing or just beyond retirement age a special deal.

The maze of details in the Social Security law, the qualification rules describing covered quarters and other technical minutia, came into play at this point. The details, for all of their fussy intricacy, provided a means of paying Social Security benefits only to those who could demonstrate a solid attachment to the labor force. To qualify for benefits under existing law, a person needed to have worked in a place covered by the program for one-half of the time between 1936 and that person's death or retirement. The intricacy of the program, however, required a series of alternatives to the rules and a number of what might be described as boundary conditions. Alternatively, a person could work in "covered employment" half of the time from age 21 to his death or retirement and still receive survivors' or old-age benefits. Someone who worked for less than six calendar quarters and then died received nothing. Someone who worked for ten years received coverage regardless of what else happened to him.

These stringent requirements rose above the marginal concerns of actuaries and others who peered at legislation from underneath a green eyeshade to concern the very essence of social policy. The rules meant that only about 20 percent of the population over 65 qualified for Social Security benefits, because someone who became 65 in 1949 would have needed six years of coverage to qualify.

To overcome these limitations, the council simply assumed them away and, tossing green eyeshades to the wind, recommended that the new people brought into the Social Security system be, in the jargon, "blanketed in." That meant changing the qualification rules for new participants to reflect, in the council's words, "previous service." Under the council's plan, the minimum of six quarters of coverage remained, but now a worker could qualify for benefits by working for half the time from the date chosen as the "new start" and the date of retirement. A regularly employed 64-year-old farm worker could work for an additional year and a half, acquiring six calendar quarters of coverage, and then retire on Social Security.

Arbitrary as these proposals appeared to be, the council refused to abandon the rules of social insurance altogether and simply pay all of the elderly a pension. "To pay benefits to all the current aged—including those who have not worked at all since the inauguration of the system—might endanger the character of the benefit based on contributions and work records," the council stated.

A final element in the effort to make Social Security strong enough to withstand the welfare challenge remained. It centered on a political accommodation of the self-employed who, many believed, held the key to the program's future. As matters stood, they remained outside of the system, neither paying taxes nor receiving benefits. That put an effective political block on ever using general revenues to fund the system because, if Congress someday decided to use general revenues, it would place the self-employed in double jeopardy, forcing them to pay Social Security taxes without providing them benefits. The self-employed, by definition, worked for themselves. That doubled their tax liability. Once again, the advisory council recommended a special deal for a politically sensitive group. This time the council decided simply to charge the self-employed less than other groups for Social Security.

Together, the council's recommendations amounted to a new start that would give social insurance parity with welfare and preserve the "contributory" nature of social insurance, but the resulting system would still contain its share of anomalies. It would not cover everyone, nor would it be totally fair in the sense that everyone received the same return on his "investment."

For all of these anomalies, the council's plan formed the basis for the 1950 amendments. Congress rewrote Social Security to the council's specifications, carping only at minor details. Some professional groups, for example, chose not to be included in the new coverage for the self-employed. When the doctors begged out, other professionals, such as undertakers, who strived for the same sort of positive image, also asked to be excluded. Congress acquiesced.

Still, a critical problem for the Social Security system lingered, just as it had since 1939. Once again, benefits were being raised and the system's future liabilities increased. In raising long-term costs, policymakers also needed to indicate some means of raising long-term revenues.

The advisory council's solution resembled earlier attempts at solving the problem. The Social Security tax rate, frozen by Congress throughout the 1940s, should finally be allowed to rise to 3 percent of payroll. In addition, the council suggested that the amount of a person's wages subject to the payroll tax be raised, thus establishing the principle that new benefits cost money, but that the next scheduled rise in the tax, to 4 percent, be postponed, thus limiting large reserves in the early years of the program. Ultimately, the council believed, the federal government should share the burden with employers and employees. Once again, therefore, an advisory group recommended that increased benefits be funded by general revenues.

Once again, Congress declined to introduce general revenues, opting instead for gradually rising tax rates. The scheduled rates began at 3 percent of payroll and would reach 6.5 percent in 1970. Congress took this action despite the fact that it had never honored previous plans to raise tax rates. Instead, it had rescinded each of the tax raises as the year they were scheduled to go into effect approached.

In deciding to take a fully funded approach, rather than to introduce general revenues, Congress argued as President Roosevelt had in 1935. The politicians believed that a contribution from general revenues, long advocated by the bureaucrats to reduce future tax rates, would be viewed as a hand-out that would send the program careening out of control. Once general revenues were introduced, said liberal New Jersey Republican Thomas Kean, an unscrupulous politician might come along and say, "I want to double that amount," and gain great advantage over responsible opponents. In this view, general revenues meant the Townsend plan redux, a bold bidding war to win the elderly's affections and political loyalty.

Kean, like his fellow legislators, understood that he was not taking much of a political risk by arguing against use of general revenues and in favor of eventually higher tax rates on employers and employees. In this case, the high moral ground also afforded firm political footing. The argument concerned the future, not the present, and, again to paraphrase Keynes, in the future we are all dead. Voters cared little about taxes in the long run, preferring to concentrate on taxes in the shorter run. Kean promised higher future taxes with every hope of not delivering them. His constituents accepted low current taxes with every hope of keeping them.

Congress, in other words, ducked the financing issue in 1950, just as it had in 1939. It allowed new benefits to begin without making any serious provision to finance them, other than to call for increased taxes in the future. As the members knew well, the future never came, and the taxes never went up, and besides, if the future should show up unannounced, it would be some other politician's problem, as indeed it was.

At the same time, the 1950 amendments represented something other than politics as usual, because by bringing social insurance to parity with welfare they changed the direction of American social policy. Congress consciously chose federally administered social insurance, despite the fact that the choice flew in the face of other trends, such as allowing the states to control and cheapen unemployment compensation and encouraging the formation of private social insurance plans.

For students of social policy, the Social Security amendments of 1950, therefore, pose a puzzle, the solution to which involves manipulating many interlocking pieces of evidence. Congress passed the 1950 amendments for reasons related to the nature of Social Security financing, partisan politics, the growth of fringe benefits, and the country's prosperity. Like other forms of social insurance legislation, the amendments appeared costless in the short run. Expansions of coverage always brought more money into the system than would have been the case without the expansion.

The timing of the amendments related to more general political events. The race with welfare became an acute problem just before the Second World War. During wartime, however, Congress hesitated to expand Social Security, and after the war, the Republicans gained control. The Republicans felt no desire to expand legislation identified as a product of the New Deal, so changes would have to wait until the Democrats resumed control of Congress in 1949. The Democratic Congress accepted both the notion of expanding Social Security and the advisory council's plan for that expansion.

The Democrats accepted the suggestions because, for the first time, the proposed amendments contained higher benefits for people in farm areas as well as in urban areas. Relatively high benefits would be paid immediately to many people in farm states who had previously been excluded from old-age insurance.

Nor did the higher benefits penalize people in the urban, industrialized sections of the country. In this respect, the growth of private social security encouraged the expansion of public social security. Business and labor leaders, faced with the costs of private pensions, began to shift some of their costs to the public sector, thereby making it easier to establish adequate pensions through collective bargaining. Older pension plans, created outside of the framework of collective bargaining agreements, provided payments that were exclusive of Social Security. Pension plans created in the 1940s in the automobile, steel, and other large industries included benefits that were inclusive of Social Security. Wilbur Cohen, the chief legislative liaison for Social Security, explained the political ramifications in a 1952 letter to one of the program's supporters. He wrote that unions were willing to go along with the "off-sets" in the newer pensions "to give employers an incentive to be in favor of increased Social Security benefits." "As you know, employers did not oppose the increased Social Security benefits in 1950 . . . and the unions claim credit for this fact."

Unions failed to rally behind expanded welfare benefits because such benefits failed to meet their needs. Someone receiving an industrial pension might not qualify for welfare. The states granted welfare as a privilege, not a right, and factory workers could not count on receiving it. Social Security came automatically, regardless of the retiree's financial condition.

In a more general sense, welfare lost some of its luster because the Depression, it was becoming increasingly clear, was over. Welfare responded to the need to help the elderly *now*, and the economy's improvement made that need less urgent. So did the fact that, under the lenient rules devised by the advisory council, members of previously excluded groups qualified quickly for Social Security.

The 1950 amendments gained acceptance also because they did not pose a direct challenge to the state welfare and unemployment compensation programs, as had earlier legislation based on the British Beveridge plan. Where the 1943 Wagner-Murray-Dingell bills proposed that the federal government take over the state unemployment compensation programs, the 1950 amendments allowed the states to continue running their unemployment compensation programs and expanded the state welfare programs by creating a completely new category of federal grants to the states, called Aid to the Permanently and Totally Disabled, and by making it easier for the states to fund the medical care of welfare recipients. As the nation would soon discover, postwar prosperity made it easier to choose among previously competing alternatives.

Each of these reasons contributed to the choice of social insurance over welfare and led to Social Security's postwar triumph. The amendments worked even better than expected. Average Social Security benefits increased by 80 percent, and in February 1951, for the first time, more people received Social Security than received old-age assistance. "We'd really crossed the mountain," said Arthur Altmeyer.

Soon Social Security had completed a reassuring transformation. A source of ideological conflict in the 1930s, it became a productive and noncontroversial program in the 1950s. In this respect, Social Security came to be perceived in a manner similar to other American institutions of the era. Neither welfare nor insurance, neither socialism nor capitalism, it represented a pragmatic middle ground, a consensus on which social policy could rest. It exemplified what some observed as America's singular ability to rise above ideology and solve social problems.

What had previously loomed as intractable issues now appeared as benign matters for experts to ponder or as accepted practices that no one bothered to challenge. In the 1950s Douglas Brown could write: "The early issue between 'pay-as-you-go' and 'large reserves' seems to have faded into the background. In old-age and survivors' insurance, we have let the actuaries worry about the problem of balancing income and outgo over time. Perhaps this is a mark of financial sophistication. We trust specialists in most aspects of life, why not in the planning of the financial aspects of social insurance?" In other words, the long-term financing of social security had moved, like other large questions of the era, beyond ideology.

Similarly, old battles between proponents of federal and state programs receded. The federal government ran old-age and survivors' insurance, the states administered unemployment compensation, and neither side seriously challenged the prerogatives of the other. Indeed, unemployment compensation, although not free from controversy, earned plaudits similar to those Social Security had begun to receive.

Contemporary authorities, who in the 1930s had regarded unemployment compensation as a dangerous drain on individual initiative, now praised the program for the way in which it stabilized the economy. When a recession hit, as it did in 1957, unemployment compensation swung into action. Just when the country appeared to be heading into a tailspin, the unemployment compensation system released money into the economy and, as economists might put it, sustained the aggregate purchasing power of consumers. President Dwight D.

Eisenhower's Council of Economic Advisers, far from disparaging the program as an unattractive remnant of the New Deal, credited unemployment compensation with preventing the 1957–58 recession from spiraling into depression. The council noted that unemployment benefits were paid in high-powered dollars that turned over a dozen times each year, compared to ordinary dollars that turned over only six times. It followed that unemployment benefit dollars were "twice as effective as any other kind of dollar." Unemployment compensation, like Social Security, had undergone a successful transformation and emerged as another quintessential modern American institution, compatible with the latest forms of Keynesian economics and the Republican politics of President Eisenhower.

Internal inconsistencies appeared not to matter in the benign light of the postwar consensus. In Social Security, for example, program features that permitted some people to receive far more for their money than did others could be dismissed as another triumph of pragmatism over hard-headed principle. Reinhard Hohaus, a private insurance actuary who had long defended the program to its private sector critics, mixed program jargon and a quintessential image of the day in his discussion of the problem: "Having concluded that both social adequacy and equity should be reflected in the old-age insurance benefit formula, the next question is how to blend the two elements. . . . Here the analogy of the best formula for a dry martini is helpful. While it seems to be generally agreed that much more gin (adequacy) should be used than vermouth (equity), there are decided differences of opinion as to what the ratio of adequacy to equity should be."

Social Security, it seemed, was as American as apple pie, as sophisticated as a dry martini, as solid as the best-run insurance company. As observers recovered their faith in the American economy, they came to see Social Security as an important component of that economy. Defending the American system of free enterprise meant defending Social Security as well.

The trouble with this view was that it assumed away fundamental problems. As early as 1960, fears of program insolvency in unemployment compensation, the result of low employer tax rates, began to spread. Self-congratulation masquerading as pragmatism carried the discussion of social policy only so far. Unless the postwar economic expansion continued forever, the bills for expanding Social Security would come due some day; and because so many people had come to depend on Social Security, the day of reckoning would be very painful for the nation's elderly citizens and for the politicians as well.

The Triumph of Social Security, 1936–1954

4   The Day of Reckoning

The economic downturn of the 1970s and 1980s produced what amounted to a major crisis in the Social Security old-age insurance program, a crisis of legitimacy that the program had not faced since the days of its race with welfare in the 1930s and the 1940s. But the program survived. The predicament ended with changes in 1983 that provided Social Security, the cornerstone of America's welfare state, with what historian W. Andrew Achenbaum has called "a new lease on life." Still, the episode left behind a bitter taste, particularly among the young, who began to examine Social Security more closely and to discover that the program depended on good economic conditions and effective political restraint for its long-range survival. The program, although in reasonably good fiscal health, became part of the crisis in the American welfare state that marked the 1970s and 1980s. By the end of the latter decade, the 1983 agreements appeared in danger of unraveling in a political environment that contained eerie resemblances to the late New Deal era at the end of the 1930s.

In the 1950s and 1960s, things had been different, and politicians had celebrated Social Security as a characteristically American institution, a marvelous mix of pluralism and pragmatism, a sure winner in Congress because of the way it transferred money to the elderly even as policymakers lauded the way it reinforced the American tradition of self-reliance.

Those decades provided ideal conditions in which to nurture a social insurance program. Wages were rising, and as they rose, more money flowed into the Social Security trust funds. Unemployment remained at low levels, meaning that money flowed into the trust funds at a steady pace. Inflation stayed low, making an investment in a long-term retirement fund appear reasonable. Fertility rates continued at high levels, insuring a high worker to beneficiary ratio far into the future as more babies grew up and had babies of their own.

Taken together, these things produced unforeseen dividends—the rewards of unexpected economic growth—that enabled the program to expand and to postpone the payment of its bills. What appeared to be long-term liabilities in 1939 and 1950 were funded through unexpected revenues that were the results of unforeseen prosperity. Although no one knew how, in the absence of general revenues or increased tax rates, the system would be able to afford such things as survivors' benefits (1939) and higher basic benefits (1950), these problems essentially solved themselves. Enough money flowed into the coffers to make general revenues or significantly higher taxes unnecessary, at least for a time.

Even during the happy days, however, the program faced potential problems. Prosperity presented a constant political temptation. Since the trust funds were chock full of money, it did not seem a disgraceful matter to vote a Social Security benefit increase, and if the increase came in an election year, well, that was simply a fortunate happenstance.

The election year ritual of Social Security benefit increases illustrated an important realignment that was occurring in pension politics. In the Depression, despite interest in the Townsend plan, much of the agitation over pensions for the elderly occurred at the state, rather than the federal, level. The pension "grabs" that occurred took place in Ohio, California, and Colorado. The emergence of Social Security changed that. Now the "gray lobby," as it came to be called, no longer concentrated on raising welfare payments or passing the Townsend Act. In the 1950s, this lobby attempted to raise Social Security benefits.

A dilemma confronted Social Security administrators. On the one hand, regular increases in social security benefits had the practical value of keeping the politicians, who sustained the program, happy. On the other hand, the practice could easily get out of control and, in the long run, undermine the program. The administrators responded to their dilemma in a practical way, encouraging the benefit increases but insisting on the integrity of their actuarial estimates as a means of setting limits. The benefit increases often took on the same ritual form as year-end corporate bonuses, something that was expected yet not guaranteed, a reward for doing a little better than had been predicted. And, if Social Security's administrators kept the predictions a little on the conservative side, with the thought of the bonus in mind, that practice harmed no one and pleased many people.

In general, Social Security administrators attempted to be responsive to the politicians, but on their own terms. Managing the program was, however, always a matter of delicate political negotiation, and the program itself was always sensitive to changes in economic conditions.

Not surprisingly, then, the economic interruption of the stagflation era of the 1970s caused trouble and strained the Social Security consensus. As prices rose faster than wages and as unemployment increased, the conditions that sustained the Social Security program began to come undone. For one thing, unemployment always posed a problem for Social Security. People who were out of work did not pay Social Security taxes, and for some of these people unemployment began a process of disengagement from the labor market that culminated in early retirement. In this manner, unemployment, doubly costly, decreased program revenues and increased program expenditures.

For another thing, a reduced standard of living caused by prices rising faster than wages made people, now accustomed to affluence, feel insecure about the future. That led some couples to have fewer children. A decline in fertility rates produced a demographic "overhang" or bulge. It meant that a large group of people would eventually have to be supported by a smaller group of people.

Finally, inflation made the program appear less attractive, as people worried that their Social Security "investment" would get eaten up by higher prices. They would contribute in hard money and receive their benefits in soft, inflated money. Saving became a less rational act in the presence of inflation, and many working Americans regarded Social Security as a form of forced savings.

Under these untoward economic conditions, people reevaluated the long-term solvency of the program and the returns on their "investments," and the Social Security consensus began to come under challenge. Characteristics once perceived as virtues became vices. Myths, tolerated by some and believed by many others, emerged as dangerous falsehoods; long-ignored contradictions, transformed into flaws, acquired a new urgency and demanded redress. The program, once regarded as carefully constructed, started to fall apart, revealing a jerry-built structure.

Over the years, for example, program administrators had skillfully managed to combine competing objectives—variously described as welfare and insurance or adequacy and equity—in one program. Such a program could be viewed either as a pragmatic triumph, as it was in the 1950s and much of the 1960s, or as an ideological muddle, as it was in the 1970s and 1980s. It was not insurance; it was not welfare.

Stagflation, by itself, would probably not have caused catastrophic trouble. The bonuses in the form of benefit increases might stop for a time, and people might grumble, but all would recognize Social Security, in the wonderfully American phrase, as a very good deal. Unfortunately, however, the bad economic conditions arose almost simultaneously with a congressional decision to grant a sharp raise in Social Security benefits. It was as if a company had decided, in one giddy moment, to take this year's bonus, next year's bonus, and the bonus for the year after that, all at once.

Then, in response, Congress compounded the problem. To protect themselves from pressures for even larger bonuses the next time around, the politicians decided to enact a fundamental "good government" reform and limit future benefit increases. That move, as it turned out, proved to be exactly wrong for the economic circumstances of the 1970s.

These actions destroyed much of the good will that the Social Security program had developed and strained the capabilities of the American political system. It took heroic efforts and unprecedented improvisation to undo the difficulties in which social security found itself.

Crisis and Response

Signs of trouble appeared within the Social Security Administration as early as 1970, when Robert J. Myers, the chief actuary, decided to resign. Internal political and personality conflicts led Myers to his decision. Myers, who was a Republican, thought that Richard Nixon, a Republican, should favor him over the incumbent Robert Ball, a Democrat, for the job of Social Security Commissioner. He thought that Ball, who had been commissioner since 1962 and who enjoyed an unexcelled reputation for administrative competence, had failed to respect the spirit and respond to the directives of the Nixon administration, just as Ball's predecessors had never really respected the desires of the Eisenhower administration. Instead, Ball and his friends had continued to operate in their usual freewheeling manner, beyond the reach of presidential politics and, in Myers's words, to "exert their efforts to expand the Social Security program as much as possible by aiding and supporting any individuals and organizations that are of this expansionist conviction."

Myers identified a major source of tension in American social policy. Simply put, the bureaucrats maintained an agenda that was

---

The Day of Reckoning

independent of the president's, and often of Congress's as well. In this case, Robert Ball, like Arthur Altmeyer before him, wanted to protect and expand the Social Security program, and he adroitly used the political situation to his advantage. Although the Republicans occupied the White House between 1969 and 1977, the Democrats controlled the Congress. Essentially, that meant that Robert Ball and his successors learned how to satisfy two masters, often by playing one against the other, while all the time speaking the language of program integrity and nonpartisan administration.

To some extent the bureaucrats consciously formulated and followed a coherent strategy; to a greater extent, however, they responded to the pressures of a policymaking environment over which they had little control. In the early days of the stagflation era, the key player in Social Security was Wilbur Mills, the chairman of the powerful House Ways and Means Committee, rather than Richard Nixon, the President of the United States. Mills, in whose committee all Social Security bills originated, made many of the final decisions about benefit increases, since it was customary for the House to debate Social Security under a closed rule that required a straight up or down vote. Although the House could approve or disapprove of a Social Security bill, it lacked the power to make substantial modifications once that bill had reached the House floor.

In 1972, Mills hoped to do something special for the program, in part because he entertained the notion of running for president. He made inquiries of Social Security officials about the possibility of an impressive benefit increase. In the end, he negotiated a spectacularly large increase of 20 percent. In order to rationalize this increase, Social Security actuaries abandoned Myers's conservative assumptions about the growth of wages. When Myers had made the actuarial estimates, he assumed that wage levels would not rise in the future and urged Congress to plan accordingly. The assumption cushioned the program against unexpected contingencies, such as sudden economic downturn. When wages rose, as they nearly always did, the surplus in social security revenues provided a welcome growth dividend that Congress always enjoyed spending. In 1972, the new actuaries, responding to pressures from economists who questioned the rationality of benefit increases funded from deliberately faulty projections, decided to do away with this safeguard. In so doing, they also managed to accommodate Mills, who wanted to use the sudden windfall for his benefit increase. Since good government and good politics appeared to coincide, the actuaries agreed to recognize the inevitability of future wage increases and to make plans for spending them. The 1972 legislation, consequently, relied on the assumption of rising wage rates as the basis for their certification as "actuarially sound."

Viewed another way, the 1972 amendments departed from the previous step-by-step approach to benefit increases and instead legislated one large benefit increase. The new approach produced the largest benefit increase in Social Security's history, raising the average level of a single retired worker's check from $133 to $166 a month.

The Republicans realized their inability to compete with a Democratic majority capable of enacting such a large benefit increase and, aware that their minority status in Congress was likely to continue, resolved to find a means of sharing the political rewards of future benefit increases. Favored by President Nixon and featured in the 1968 Republican platform, the chosen vehicle clothed a political objective in the uplifting rhetoric of sound governmental practice. The Republicans, urging policymakers to put future benefit increases on a more scientific, less partisan basis, advocated a change known as "indexing." Replacing congressional action each election year, indexing would mean automatic adjustments in benefit levels, based on changes in the consumer price index. Benefits would, beginning in 1975, keep pace with the inflation rate as measured by the consumer price index.

Indexing represented a new way of raising Social Security benefits that many people, inside bureaucrats and outside critics, Republicans and Democrats, believed superior to the old way of regularly spending unexpected surpluses. In 1972, therefore, Congress took one last growth dividend—giving Mills what he wanted—and simultaneously shifted over to the new system—providing the administration with what it wanted. Congress tucked indexing and the benefit increase into a veto-proof measure to raise the public debt limit and passed it in July.

Another fateful change occurred in 1972, as a result of President Nixon's welfare reform efforts. Congress enacted the Supplemental Security Income (SSI) program, which was scheduled to go into effect in 1974. This program not only provided a guaranteed income to the needy elderly, blind, and disabled, it also included an administrative shift in these programs. Traditionally run as welfare programs by the states, these programs would now be administered by the federal government, with the Social Security Administration as the responsible agent.

These two major pieces of legislation led to financial and administrative crises. Economic conditions put unexpected pressure on the Social Security program at a time when the margin for error had been reduced by the changes in actuarial assumptions and the large benefit increases already legislated. The administrative demands of implementing new programs such as SSI tarnished the Social Security Administration's reputation for excellence. Late in November 1975, for example, a House committee reporting on the SSI program noted "unacceptable delays," "errors in payments," and a failure to "enroll up to 2 million eligible individuals."

This administrative failure resulted partly from the distractions caused by the financing issues that had begun to dominate the Social Security agenda by 1975. The actuaries in charge of overseeing the old-age, survivors' and disability insurance trust funds reported that the program faced critical financing problems. If nothing were done, the program would run out of money. Such reports heightened fears among the young that their Social Security investments were not safe; and program supporters, such as Robert Ball, realized that the support of the young was critical to the future of the program.

In 1977, Congress intervened to shore up the program's finances. Amendments in that year included a new benefit formula that had the effect of reducing benefit levels. Other changes involved a rise in the amount of a person's wages that was subject to Social Security taxes, with provisions for a formula that would automatically adjust the "maximum taxable earnings" in the future. Most importantly, the amendments provided for increased tax rates, which were scheduled to reach 7.65 percent on employers and employees by 1990.

Even with these adjustments, financial problems continued. The culprit was the economy. In 1978, actuaries assumed that wages would increase faster than prices. They predicted a "real wage differential" (the difference between the percentage increase in average annual wages and the percentage increase in the average annual Consumer Price Index) of 2.2 in 1980. The actual figure was -4.5. That meant that the ratio of program expenditures to program revenues increased much faster than expected, leading to another crisis. In 1981, the year President Jimmy Carter left office, officials estimated that, without further action, Social Security would run out of money in a few years. Reacting to this news, a majority of people began to believe that Social Security would not be there for them when they retired. The day of reckoning, so long postponed, now appeared to be at hand.

Many people, particularly those on the political right, stepped up their attacks on Social Security. In the view of analysts in such places as the Cato Institute and the Heritage Foundation, Social Security was a shell game that could not be sustained indefinitely. At first, small numbers of beneficiaries received windfall gains from large numbers of contributors. The apparent financial soundness of the program emboldened the beneficiaries to seek even larger benefits. Contributors failed to object because taxes remained low. Eventually, however, demographic realities caught up with the program, the ratio of contributors to beneficiaries began to fall, and windfall gains became no longer possible. Conservative analysts believed it was time for politicians to be honest with the people and to convert the program into what the Heritage Foundation called an "actuarially sound" annuity program, in which people received only what they had "earned." Such a move would put the public and private sectors on a more equal footing and pave the way for a voluntary system of social security.

Between 1964 and 1980, the notion of abandoning the present Social Security system and converting it to a voluntary system came out of the closet. When Senator Barry Goldwater, running as the Republican candidate for president in 1964, raised the possibility of making Social Security voluntary, he damaged his political reputation perhaps irrevocably. The Democrats, reported journalist Teddy White, chose to hang Goldwater "on one issue: Social Security." President Lyndon Johnson, mercilessly exploiting Goldwater's apparent inability to appreciate the complexities of modern life, pilloried Goldwater on Social Security. The issue remained taboo politically for the next sixteen years; and even Ronald Reagan, whose national political roots went back to the Goldwater campaign and who articulated the new conservative vision as effectively as any American politician, stayed away from it. At the same time, it became, if not possible for presidential candidates to discuss the issue, somewhat more respectable for other politicians to point out the program's shortcomings. For the young, a voluntary system presented the increasingly attractive option of leaving a program that reduced their take home pay without, if the prophets of doom were to be believed, increasing their retirement income.

Once safely in office, Ronald Reagan, whose administration made considerable use of the Heritage Foundation's suggestions, contemplated fundamental reform of Social Security. In May 1981, administration officials unveiled a benefit reduction package that was their response to the financial crisis. The package included reductions in benefits for people who retired at age 62 and a six-month delay in making the required benefit adjustments to reflect increases in the price of living. The rationale for the proposed changes was simple and direct. As budget director David Stockman noted, the program would go bankrupt by October 1982 without such changes.

Reagan's initiative failed to fly. Congress objected, and loudly. What most disturbed the congressmen was that the administration wanted to change the rules without giving people due warning. The Senate quickly passed a resolution to that effect, saying, for example, that "Congress shall not precipitously and unfairly reduce early retirees' benefits." Once again, a Republican politician learned the political potency of the Social Security issue.

Despite posturing on both sides, Social Security faced a deep crisis, and something needed to be done about it. Congress made small, incremental changes in Social Security, but they were not nearly enough. In July 1981, for example, Congress agreed to such measures as the elimination of student benefits for people aged 18–21. Unappeased, conservatives continued to speak of necessary fundamental reforms. Liberals argued that the conservatives were using a temporary crisis—that would almost certainly right itself in the 1990s, when large Social Security surpluses would appear, and could therefore easily be solved by temporarily borrowing money from general revenues—as a means of destroying America's most successful social program.

Frustrated by the congressional reaction, Reagan administration officials proposed the creation of a presidential commission to study the problem. The president appointed the National Commission on Social Security Reform on December 16, 1981. If nothing else, it served as a means of getting the administration through the 1982 elections. When someone asked president Reagan about Social Security, he could reply that he was waiting for the commission's report before taking action.

The membership of the commission differed from that of previous Social Security advisory councils in that it included prominent politicians and inside players, rather than the usual assortment of distinguished individuals representing the interests of labor, management, and the general public. The president, the Republican congressional leadership, and the Democratic congressional leadership each named five members. The membership included Senator Robert Dole, a potential presidential candidate and the chairman of the Senate Finance Committee, Senator John Heinz, the liberal Republican in charge of the Senate Special Committee on Aging, New York's Senator Daniel Moynihan, Representative Barber Conable, who was the ranking Republican on the House Ways and Means Committee, and Claude Pepper, the leading advocate on behalf of the elderly in Congress. In addition, Robert Ball, the former Commissioner of Social Security who continued to be exceptionally active in program politics, served as a member, and Robert Myers, the former social security actuary, directed the commission's staff. Economist Alan Greenspan chaired the commission.

The Social Security Crisis

Expectations for the commission were nonetheless low. No one fully expected the commissioners to cut a deal that would be acceptable to both the president and the Democratic leadership in the House of Representatives. Each side profoundly mistrusted the other. The Democrats worried that the Republicans would "oversolve" the problem and make unnecessary benefit cuts. The Republicans worried that the Democrats would fail to come to grips with the problem and continue to use Social Security as a campaign issue against the Republicans.

The president subscribed to this general wisdom, realizing that appointing a commission conformed to the standard political ploy of sidestepping a troublesome problem. As president Reagan should have understood, however, Social Security, unlike pension reform or biomedical ethics, for example, had traditionally used advisory councils to confront difficult political issues. Robert Ball, the staff director of the 1948 advisory council, and Robert Myers, the actuary for all of the advisory councils going back to 1938, respected this tradition and wished to preserve it. And this commission, unlike previous advisory councils, contained more than its share of practical politicians, whose presence almost guaranteed that discussions of fundamental reform, such as President Reagan might have favored, would be short and preemptory. Instead, the discussions would take place with an eye toward the immediate political situation, well within the contours of the possible.

Robert Ball, for one, never dismissed the hope that the commission could reach an agreement. He was extremely worried about the program's future and hoped, as he put it, to get the Social Security program off the front pages for the next fifty years. When he met with Alan Greenspan for breakfast in the Watergate Hotel early in January 1982, for example, he stressed the need not to get bogged down in philosophical issues and instead to concentrate on a practical solution. Throughout the long commission meetings, Ball maintained the emphasis on pragmatic, nonideological measures, portraying the problem as one of coming up with money in the short run rather than as one that required fundamental changes in the program itself. Ball also insisted on limiting the discussion to the financing issue, rather than broadening it to include such matters as health insurance.

As Ball and others realized, however, coming up with money involved both technical and political decisions. Given the choice, conservatives favored cutting back on benefits and liberals preferred raising taxes. Ball and others searched for sources of revenue that were not neatly categorized as a benefit cut or a tax increase. They found two major items. Extending coverage, the first item, cleverly increased program revenues without raising taxes. Taxing the benefits of upper-income people, the second item, served either as a cut in benefits or an increase in taxes, a very useful ambiguity.

Each of these things reflected the peculiar economics of Social Security. Expanding coverage created the same situation as had existed in 1935. Because of the pay and play rule, members of the newly covered group would, for many years to come, pay in far more than they would get back. Hence, in the immediate political context, an extension of coverage raised revenues. Similarly, taxing Social Security benefits could be put to many useful purposes. Under the proper conditions, it provided a disguised way to realize long-held ambitions and introduce general revenues into the program. Accomplishing this objective required a simple rule not to dump the taxes collected on Social Security benefits into the treasury but instead to dedicate this money for Social Security's use. Nor did the political attractiveness of the measure stop there. Taxing benefits for people with high incomes neatly separated key supporters from others with less enthusiasm for the program. The measure preserved the system and retained present benefits for the broad middle class, including members of organized labor, whose benefits, presumably, would not be taxed.

The commission met nine times in 1982, waiting for the election to be over and holding informational seminars on the nature of Social Security. Ball spent this time contributing to the huge pool of memoranda that the commission and staff director Myers were generating, and meeting with the Democratic commissioners. In June, Ball held a long discussion with commission member Lane Kirkland, the head of the American Federation of Labor–Congress of Industrial Organizations (AFL-CIO), probing acceptable bargaining positions. That same month, Ball wrote a report on why Individual Retirement Accounts (IRAs) were not an acceptable substitute for Social Security. That summer, the commission itself heard a long lecture by Robert Myers on how the monies in the Social Security trust funds were invested and attended a seminar on the economics of Social Security, jointly conducted by Michael Boskin, a spokesman for the conservative side and later the chairman of President Bush's Council of Economic Advisers, and Henry Aaron, a spokesman for the liberal side and a former official in the Carter administration.

Listening to Boskin, Joe Waggoner, a former congressman and a conservative, responded that the commission did not want to re-do the Social Security system so much as it wanted to concentrate on the immediate financing problem. Ball could not have been more pleased.

The 1982 elections made the Republicans realize just how bad an

The Social Security Crisis

issue Social Security was for them. The Democrats gained seats in Congress, in part because people feared that the Republicans would somehow jeopardize their Social Security benefits.

After the election, serious negotiations began. The first postelection meeting took place in Alexandria, Virginia. Ball had insisted that before the meeting the commission staff prepare a book that listed all of the possible alternatives for restoring Social Security's financial integrity. He encouraged people to put together different alternatives in order to come up with an acceptable plan. The very presence of the book took some of the ideological edge off the discussion and forced the commissioners to think in pragmatic terms.

The meeting in Alexandria resulted in the commission's first major agreement. The commissioners voted to accept a figure on the size of the short-term and long-term Social Security deficit. The commission, in effect, agreed not to fight over the severity of the problem and instead to accept the estimate that $150–$200 billion would be needed between 1983 and 1989. For the long term, the commission members concurred in a deficit that, in the Social Security tradition, was expressed as a percentage of taxable payroll. In this case, the size of the long-range deficit was 1.8 percent of taxable payroll. That meant that, in the long run, taxes would have to be raised by this amount to cover the deficit and have the system break even.

The need to vote on these figures underscored how even questions of fact were subject to differing political interpretations. Each side had been burned by recent events. The 1977 experience had made a great impression on the Democrats. What at the time had seemed an adequate solution turned out to be inadequate. Few of the commissioners, and certainly not the Democratic commissioners, wanted to repeat 1977 and reach a deal that became unstuck because of unexpected economic forces. To accept a high target figure provided protection against such a development. The Democrats also realized that a higher target increased the pressure on the Republicans to support higher taxes. The Democrats already enjoyed reasonable protection against what they regarded as excessive benefit cuts, since the president, mindful of his 1981 experience, had pledged not to cut the value of benefits for people already receiving them and had learned that the program could not be changed without due notice. That limited the changes that could be made in the critical period between 1983 and 1989.

As for the longer-term estimates, the Commission made what amounted to a deal within a deal. The Democrats wanted the actuaries to bless the commission's work and, to gain that blessing, agreed to the actuaries' long-range estimates of Social Security's deficits. In return, the Republicans agreed not to push the conservative line that the long-range estimates understated the severity of the problem.

As the commissioners took these steps in public, meetings occurred in private on the possibility of an agreement. Ball spoke to Robert Dole about whether the Senator would be interested in a concession from the Democrats that went beyond the three-month delay in the cost of living adjustment to which the Democrats had already agreed. Dole, who, like Ball, saw the practical advantage in the commission's coming to agreement, reacted with interest. Informal discussions then began with Greenspan, who passed along word to the White House that the Democrats might be willing to make further concessions.

In December, Ball continued his meetings with his fellow Democratic commissioners and held confidential meetings with White House officials. Agreement, however, seemed out of reach. The White House officials and Greenspan could not, for example, understand Ball's reluctance to agree to raising the retirement age. Ball replied that a higher retirement age would mean asking people to pay higher rates and then get fewer years of benefits. Furthermore, in a time of high unemployment, people would not be receptive to proposals for raising the retirement age. Also, in general, attitudes toward work differed between white and blue collar workers; blue collar workers placed less emphasis on work as a means of self-fulfillment than did white collar workers and consequently valued retirement more. Viewing the higher retirement age as a betrayal, blue collar workers might take out their political frustrations on the Democratic politicians whom they traditionally supported.

Beyond this matter, differences between the two sides over how to meet the long-term and short-term deficits persisted. The White House officials sincerely believed, that, in the long run, the scope of the program needed to be cut back. The Democrats equally sincerely felt that, in the long run, the scope of the program should remain the same. Impasse loomed.

Then, unexpectedly, a breakthrough occurred in January 1983. Senator Dole published an op-ed piece in the *New York Times* in which he stated that the problem could be solved through some combination of benefit cuts and tax increases. Senator Moynihan, who was plunged into despair over the inability of the political system to cope with Social Security, responded favorably to Dole's piece and approached him about extending the negotiations. Moynihan, who realized the need for technical help and political guidance, brought in Ball, and the three of them brought in Barber Conable and Alan

The Social Security Crisis

Greenspan. This group largely took it upon itself to meet with James Baker, the White House chief of staff (and later President Bush's secretary of state).

Each of the participants in the negotiations viewed the problem in the pragmatic terms favored by Ball, whose desire to preserve the program was paramount. Dole, for his part, continued to see the agreement as important to his future, and Moynihan wanted to demonstrate the capacity of the system to govern. Each of these people, and Conable and Greenspan and Baker as well, wanted to find a solution.

At some point in January, the White House came to understand that Robert Ball and Claude Pepper might agree to a six-month delay in the cost of living adjustment, and that proved to be the crucial breakthrough. It meant that current beneficiaries would have to wait longer to receive their benefit increases and, in effect, that their total benefits from Social Security would be permanently reduced, since that money would never be made up. It was as though a bank decided to wait six months before paying interest in a bank account. The total savings attributed to this measure were $40 billion between 1983 and 1989. Negotiators matched this figure with $40 billion worth of tax increases. The negotiators added extensions of coverage and other technical items and came up with a package that would produce $168 billion between 1983 and 1989.

By Saturday, January 15, 1983, a compromise agreement was in place, and members of the bargaining party began to contact other commissioners to see whether they could support it. Robert Ball, calling from Blair House, the president's guest quarters located across the street from the White House, telephoned Lane Kirkland, the head of the AFL-CIO, who had just returned from a speech in New York. He called Speaker of the House Tip O'Neill, who was in a West Coast hotel getting ready to play in a celebrity golf tournament. He called Claude Pepper. Although it took varying degrees of persuasion, all three agreed to the compromise.

At seven in the evening, David Stockman, Richard Darman, Jim Baker, and other White House officials walked across the street from the west wing of the White House and said that President Reagan would agree to the deal if the Democrats would. The commission soon formally accepted the agreement by a 12-3 vote.

On January 25, 1983, Robert Ball received a call from President Reagan congratulating him on the commission's work. The president praised the commission for demonstrating that bipartisan government could function effectively. A week before, Moynihan had made the same point in a *Washington Post* op-ed piece headed "More than

Social Security Was at Stake." "There is a center in American government. It can govern," wrote Moynihan.

The Compromise in Congress

All of those associated with the commission's work emphasized that the compromise must stand or fall as a package. If the package came undone, both sides would run for political cover and the measure would fail. Wilbur Cohen, a former secretary of Health, Education, and Welfare, a long-time Washington insider on Social Security and head of an organization called Save Our Security, understood this fact and put his blessing on the compromise. However, the American Association of Retired Persons, a key faction of the gray lobby, protested vigorously against the delay in the cost of living adjustment. Federal employee groups, whose future members would be required to join the Social Security program as part of the extension of coverage, also raised objections.

Meanwhile, a dispute developed over how best to deal with the long-range deficit. The commission had left about a third of the long-range deficit "unsolved," in order, in Barber Conable's phrase, "to give Danny Rostenkowski (the chairman of the Ways and Means Committee) something to sink his teeth into." It was, in other words, up to Congress, rather than the commission, to make the final cuts or tax increases that would put the program into balance for the foreseeable future. Unfortunately, Congress was bitterly divided on the issue.

One congressional faction, headed by Representative "Jake" Pickle, a Democrat from the Texas hill country near Austin, wanted to raise the retirement age for the baby boom generation and in this way lower the system's future liabilities. Another faction, headed by Claude Pepper, a Democrat from a retirement-laden district in southern Florida, vigorously opposed this measure and favored additional tax raises to make up the long-range deficit, should such taxes prove necessary. This approach incorporated the familiar postponement strategy that had proved so successful in the past.

Despite these disagreements, the measure passed, and passed quickly. Introduced in January, the 1983 amendments became law by April. The completed amendments included the provision for raising the retirement age to 67 in the next century. In other words, they followed the lead of Representative Pickle rather than that of Representative Pepper. Otherwise, they very closely resembled the commission plan.

Congress acted with such dispatch because it was mindful that, without some sort of action, the system would go bankrupt by mid-year. The media continually emphasized this point. *Newsweek*, in a cautious story about the commission agreement that stressed the intergenerational tensions within the Social Security program, reported that without an agreement, "the checks owed to 36 million retirees on July 3 would simply not be mailed."

It was an extraordinary performance: a serious political negotiation to cope with the cost pressures on a social welfare program, a successful exercise in what political scientist Martha Derthick has called "the politics of subtraction." The commission's success hinged on the considerable talents of individuals, such as Robert Ball, Robert Myers, and Alan Greenspan, who managed to find common ground when the task had seemed impossible.

At the same time, the commission owed its success to the limited way in which it defined the problem. It did not reform the American social welfare system or the American approach to old-age policy or even the American retirement system. Instead, it made some adjustments to a program that people in the political center agreed was important to preserve. Accomplishing even this goal required improvising a new set of institutional arrangements, to remove the problem from the immediate attention of Congress.

Of course, these arrangements were not entirely improvised and not entirely new. Social Security had always depended on outside management and on negotiations conducted outside of Congress in order to succeed. The commission widened the process to include White House and congressional representatives and, in the end, both of these political players came to see the value in a negotiated settlement over a full-scale political donnybrook conducted in Congress. The Democrats worried, for example, that they might not be able to produce a congressional agreement. As it was, the process exposed tensions between Representatives Pickle and Pepper, and the Senate side of the Congress was in Republican hands. The Republicans simply did not trust Congress to produce an acceptable plan.

Social Security and the Crisis of the Welfare State

Contrary to the expectations of President Roosevelt and his advisors, the Social Security system failed to become self-supporting; it failed to make adequate provisions for its future. The system never escaped the political pressures from which Brown, Armstrong, and Latimer hoped to protect it. Somewhere along the line, politicians derailed the program and turned it into another social benefit, subject to political negotiation.

Viewed another way, Social Security also proved to be highly enduring, preserved by careful thought and careless luck. The notion of an implied contract between the workers and the government enabled the program to achieve a respectability and level of participation that was unprecedented in American history. The postwar economy made it possible for the program to escape the dilemmas in which politicians had put it in 1939 and 1950. Demography and economics caught up with the program, but the process took a long time; and even then, the program had acquired the necessary good will that allowed it to survive.

The postwar consensus, however, no longer governs the program. The American voting public no longer approaches the program with the willing suspension of disbelief that, in the past, induced the feeling that the future somehow takes care of itself. The public now knows that responsible policymakers have, despite their considerable expertise, led the program into a state of financial crisis and that these same policymakers have produced reforms that have postponed, rather than eliminated further crisis. Such knowledge leads to the bitter sense that the program may be beyond rescue and undermines support for the very foundation on which the entire American welfare state rests.

The Social Security program has come full circle, from crisis, to consensus, and back to crisis. Even the work of the 1983 commission served only to complete the loop, because the future solvency of Social Security now rests on assumptions similar to those made by President Roosevelt in 1935.

Social Security's defenders, such as Robert Ball, claim that the program should be solvent through the year 2050. The claim rests on elaborate plans to fund the retirement of the baby boom generation by building up a surplus through the year 2030. The proposal follows the consequences of the population's age structure. In the 1930s, the depressed state of the economy caused the birth rate to fall; those born in that decade will reach the prime retirement age of 65 between 1995 and 2005. High tax rates, paid by members of the large postwar cohorts, combined with gently increasing Social Security beneficiary rolls will produce a surplus. The size of this surplus remains an educated guess. If one looks at the 1985 projections, one finds a drop in the cost of Social Security benefits from 11.3 percent of payroll in 1985 to 10.2 percent in 2004. Whatever the exact size of the surplus, it appears almost certain to develop.

The official version of what should happen emphasizes the continued growth of the trust funds through the years in which the baby boom generation will be retiring. Someone born in 1950 who retires at the new regular retirement age of 67 will become eligible for regular Social Security benefits in 2017. By 2035, when the bulk of the baby boom will have retired, Social Security costs should reach 15.5 percent of payroll. By then, however, the system should have begun to spend the considerable surplus from a trust fund projected to reach $12 trillion in 2030.

The official plan presupposes the orderly growth of the Social Security surplus through the willingness of the public to bear higher tax rates and the ability of the government to invest the surplus in a way that preserves the money for future generations. Indeed, the plan closely resembles President Roosevelt's original plan, with only the magnitude of the numbers changed. A $47 billion surplus, envisioned in the New Deal, has grown into the currently contemplated multitrillion-dollar surplus.

Since political and economic circumstances defeated President Roosevelt's plan, one wonders about the prospects for the 1983 plan. Will fate be kinder to President Reagan's Social Security reforms than to President Roosevelt's? The answer appears to be no. Already events have cast doubt on the scheme's ability to fund the baby boom's retirement, as the capitol intrigues of 1989 indicated.

Ronald Reagan left office in 1989 proud of his efforts to reduce taxes, yet the record showed the less-than-complete nature of his triumph. As Paul Gigot of the *Wall Street Journal* noted, the share of the economy represented by federal taxes remained the same throughout the 1980s. Income taxes declined, but payroll taxes, such as Social Security, easily made up the difference.

Even as the departing president safely settled in on easy street, his Social Security taxes put in place by the 1977 amendments kept on generating more and more revenue. In January 1990, for example, workers discovered larger Social Security deductions in their paychecks, as the employee's share increased from 7.51 to 7.65 percent of "taxable" wages (for Old-Age, Survivors', and Disability Insurance). "No new taxes. Who says so?" asked the *Boston Globe*. Social Security taxes now took an undeniably healthy bite out of workers' earnings. If one also counted the employer's contribution that might otherwise have increased their wages, nearly three-quarters of those who contributed to Social Security paid more in Social Security taxes than in income taxes.

President George Bush took office in 1989 determined to reduce the size of the national debt. Aware of the extraordinary economic pressures on the federal budget, Bush welcomed any means of lowering the debt, any source of revenue that could be counted against the deficit. Social Security taxes, being collected from nearly everyone and yielding impressive surpluses, immediately popped into mind. They produced a cool $52 billion in 1989 that could be used to offset a portion of the deficit. Social Security funds lowered the deficit from $204 to $152 billion.

Concerned about the debt, President Bush nonetheless made a pledge not to raise taxes. "Read my lips," he told a national television audience, "No new taxes." The president even entertained the notion of a tax reduction, focusing on the capital gains tax that, he argued, discouraged investment and reduced America's ability to compete in the global economy.

Senator Daniel Patrick Moynihan saw an opportunity to teach President George Bush a political lesson. A veteran of the 1983 commission, Moynihan had worried for years about Social Security's inability to sustain a surplus in a time of budgetary deficit. He saw the situation of the 1980s in exactly the same way as Senator Vandenberg had seen the 1930s. The government took the Social Security money and neither saved nor invested it but spent it. As the Republicans had expressed the idea in their 1936 platform, "the so-called reserve fund . . . is no reserve at all, because the fund will contain nothing but the government's promise to pay, while the taxes collected in the guise of premiums will be wasted in reckless and extravagant political schemes." Said Moynihan, "There is a word for this. The word is *thievery.*"

In December 1989, Moynihan resolved to make good on his previous threats and to call a halt to the plans for a Social Security surplus. His previous role as a creator of the 1983 amendments lent authority to his efforts, as did his unquestioned support for Social Security. On December 29, Moynihan announced that he would sponsor legislation to repeal the Social Security tax increase scheduled to begin on January 1 and to restore Social Security financing to a pay-as-you-go basis by reducing future Social Security tax rates. Having dropped his bomb, Moynihan departed, in a manner reminiscent of President Theodore Roosevelt, for Africa.

The story played on the inside of most newspapers. The *Washington Post*, for example, ran it on page six. Then, reaction began to build, as the media focused more attention on the proposal during the domestic news shortage that often develops during the holiday season. This was the time for slower, less dramatic, more reflective stories to appear. In this particular case, the story also related to a number of timely themes, such as the true meaning of the Reagan years now that Reagan's decade was ending, the significance of a growing federal debt, and the fate of the baby boom in the next century. The follow-stories played lead through the holiday season and into January as a new congressional session approached.

These news stories and commentaries bore a close resemblance to the stories about President Roosevelt's plans for a Social Security reserve. Spencer Rich, of the *Washington Post*, wrote of a "mountain of money growing in Washington. . . . But—as happens in Washington—the mountain isn't exactly a mountain, and the money isn't exactly money." As the Republicans had said in 1936, "the reserve is no reserve at all." Thomas Sowell, the black conservative economist and syndicated columnist, called attention to the use of Social Security taxes to fund regular governmental activities. "If you watched the astronauts in space or the American troops in Panama," he wrote, "you were seeing your Social Security dollars at work." Perhaps Sowell had stolen a glance at a Mark Sullivan column from the 1930s in which Sullivan wrote on how Social Security revenues paid the government's current bills, "perhaps to finance WPA projects in street paving, perhaps to pay the salaries of officers in the Navy."

Politicians, avid readers of the opinion columns, scrambled for cover in the face of a proposed tax cut that contrasted nicely with the president's proposal for a cut in the capital gains tax. One helped the middle classes; the other aided the rich. Seldom in recent years had the Democrats been able to cast political alternatives in such attractive terms. One White House official confided, "You've got normal people who are tired of Social Security. You've got businesses that are tired of paying Social Security, and you've got an election year. You've got a match, and you've got gasoline."

Moynihan's measure even divided the Social Security insiders. Robert Myers, who had helped to write the proposal, lent Moynihan his support; Robert Ball opposed Moynihan. Myers's argument read as though he had consulted a textbook from the 1930s. Surpluses, he said, created "irresistible pressure" for liberalization that could "not readily be undone when the baby boomers retire." He continued to favor a pay-as-you-go plan that harkened back to the step-by-step planning for Social Security that had characterized his tenure as chief actuary. Robert Ball opposed the Moynihan proposal, arguing the need for a larger reserve in 1990, to provide a cushion against an unexpected economic downturn or financing problems that might develop in the Medicare (health insurance) program.

Even Ball, however, signaled a willingness to back away from the 1983 accords and the method of surplus financing, once the program developed a "safer reserve." Ball agreed with economist Henry Aaron of the Brookings Institution, who pegged the success of a Social Security surplus to raising the "level of overall savings now, making more money available for investment to promote future growth." Both

The Day of Reckoning

Ball and Aaron understood that Social Security revenues used to invade Panama, pay interest on the national debt, or bail out bankrupt savings and loans failed to accomplish this purpose. "A Social Security build-up that increases our capacity to produce is theoretically possible but not easy to accomplish," wrote Ball. The Long Island tabloid *Newsday* explained the problem in simpler terms, "Social Security is in trouble because it has too much money while the rest of the government continues to have far too little."

All in all, history provides little encouragement to people who have rational plans for the future of Social Security, yet history also shows how unreliable the past can be as a guide to the future in this matter. Although the plans of Social Security's founders did not work out, the program still managed to thrive in the period from 1950 until 1975.

In the end, Social Security depends on public confidence. The critical problem concerns the young. The elderly have every reason to support Social Security. They either benefit directly or can look forward to a day when they will. The young have less reason to believe in the eventual existence of retirement benefits. The program's more immediate benefits, such as death or disability benefits, either fail to register or are simply too painful to contemplate. How many young people give even passing consideration to the economic burden lifted from their shoulders by having their parents and grandparents on Social Security? Hence, young people's feelings about Social Security depend solely on their perceptions of its long-term solvency.

Despite reassurances from authorities, the young continue to remain skeptical. Many who have watched the real Social Security crises of the 1970s and the 1980s unfold feel that the program has something of a permanent taint. Social Security's situation resembles that of the beleaguered savings and loan industry, which once thrived, lending people money to buy houses but found itself caught by the rising interest rates of the 1970s. As the S and L's, trapped between the low interest on their mortgages and the high interest demanded by investors, began to lose money, people hesitated to bank with them, demonstrating that whatever other problems an institution might face, a lack of confidence is crippling in and of itself. In the case of the thrifts, people had choices and exercised them. In the end, the government needed to come to the rescue of the savings and loan industry. In the case of Social Security, people have fewer choices—they must participate—but they can begin to create a political climate hospitable to new alternatives, such as making Social Security voluntary for the young.

Defenders of Social Security, who correctly perceive calls to make

Social Security voluntary as death threats, work to shore up confidence. They believe that the barbarians, intent upon destroying America's most successful social welfare program and bringing down the entire American welfare state, are at the gates. As a result, they spend little time making changes in the program to reflect modern realities. One wonders, for example, if the retirement age should not be raised further to reflect trends in health and in the desires of the elderly: maybe the elderly want to work but, finding the loss of their Social Security benefits too much of a penalty to bear, instead decide to retire. Social Security no longer faces the problems of the 1930s, when it was imperative that the elderly retire. One also wonders about the continuing system of paying everyone a Social Security benefit: maybe the affluent do not need Social Security and would be willing to do without it or pay higher taxes on the benefits that they do receive.

Raising the retirement age and changing the fundamental rules of Social Security entitlement remain highly controversial matters. The relevant point, however, is that the present crisis atmosphere provides no opportunities for these matters to be discussed. Defenders of Social Security are too busy assuring everyone that it remains a good deal; opponents of Social Security are too busy trying to prove that sleight of hand cannot be sustained indefinitely. Stifling creative discussion, the crisis of the welfare state that began with the economic downturn of the 1970s continues to impose its costs on the nation.

★ ★ ★

II

The Frustrations of Welfare Reform

5   Welfare's State, 1935–1967

In 1935, President Franklin D. Roosevelt hoped, against considerable odds, that social insurance might eventually emerge as the primary solution to the nation's social welfare problems. If Roosevelt had lived beyond 1945, he would have seen Social Security's 1950 triumph fulfill his hopes. Roosevelt took as his major premise the corrosive effects of welfare on the human spirit, its effect as a narcotic, and saw in social insurance an uplifting rather than soul-destroying program. Between 1935 and 1965, a dichotomy between the two approaches developed: social insurance paid people for working; welfare encouraged people not to work. Hence, the substitution of social insurance for welfare became an important priority of social policy.

During the years of the midcentury social welfare consensus, presidents from Harry Truman to Gerald Ford proclaimed the virtues of social insurance. At the heart of this consensus lay an idealized picture of a person who maintained a steady relationship with both his employer and the state. Most people worked or, in the case of women, children, and handicapped adults, depended on someone who worked. Workers supplied their families with a current source of income and, cooperating with employers and government, saved money to meet adverse contingencies, such as unemployment, disability, and ill health. As they protected themselves against these unfortunate events, they also contributed regularly to a retirement fund, backed by the government's financial integrity, that guaranteed a source of income and shielded them from crippling medical expenses from the day they retired to the day they died.

Roosevelt regarded welfare as a narcotic, to which people became addicted, yet he endorsed it as a political necessity. Even though the president vowed in 1935 to remove the federal government from the "business of relief," he supported legislation that granted money to the states for welfare. In so doing, he paved the way for a great irony of social policy history. The program designed to take the government out of the relief business proved to be the one that established the modern welfare system.

In proposing the Social Security Act, President Roosevelt honored an important distinction between *relief* and *pensions*. *Relief* meant temporary aid for people of working age; *pensions* implied permanent payments for people unable to work. Roosevelt wanted to get the government out of the relief business and initiate an orderly transfer of pensions from welfare to social insurance and from the states to the federal government. He therefore replaced the dole with a public works program that made work a condition for the receipt of benefits. He also initiated a social insurance program and, only as an interim measure during the initial years of the social insurance program, agreed to reimburse the states for part of the costs of pensions.

In the president's view, not everyone deserved a pension. Instead, the Social Security Act established strict eligibility categories. Only people who were old and out of work, young and deprived of parental support, or blind and incapacitated qualified for a state administered but federally assisted pension. Others in need of aid would have to depend on the far less certain generosity of state and local programs, called "general assistance," that lacked recourse to federal funds.

In the beginning, welfare fared better than social insurance. The ideological battles and political confrontations that marked the first fifteen years of Social Security's history did not apply to welfare. Instead, policymakers accepted welfare either as a transitional device necessary until social insurance took hold or as a program superior to social insurance that targeted money for those who needed it the most, reinforced local government's responsibility to aid the poor, and limited payments to the precise period of need. Either way, welfare in the form of pensions enjoyed widespread approval.

The triumph of Social Security indicated the successful transition from welfare pensions to social insurance pensions. In 1939, survivors' benefits allowed social insurance to pay benefits to widows and dependent children, lessening the need for state pensions for dependent children. Between 1940 and 1945 and again between 1950 and 1955, the average monthly number of families on Aid to Dependent Children (ADC or, after 1962, AFDC) fell. In 1950, expanded coverage and higher Social Security benefit levels eliminated much of the need for state welfare pensions for the elderly. Beginning in 1950, the average monthly number of recipients of old-age assistance declined steadily from year to year.

Despite these encouraging trends, the federal government never left the relief business. By the end of the 1950s, policymakers grudgingly recognized the existence of a welfare problem because Aid to Families with Dependent Children never faded away, even as the social insurance program grew. Instead, AFDC changed from a respectable pension program into a dole with growing costs and a growing caseload. AFDC payments replaced general assistance aimed more generally at the poor and emerged in the 1950s as America's major welfare program. In 1936, for example, eight times as many people obtained general assistance, the traditional relief programs funded by the states and localities, as received Aid to Dependent Children, the new pension program funded by the states and the federal government. In 1975, the number of general assistance beneficiaries stood below the 1936 level, and the AFDC caseload exceeded the general assistance caseload by a factor of twelve. Despite high levels of economic growth, declining barriers to women's participation in the labor force, and the extraordinary rise in social insurance payments, the AFDC rolls rose from 3 million people in an average month in 1960, to 4.3 million in 1965, to 8.5 million in 1970, and to 11.3 million in 1975. President Roosevelt never envisioned that.

By the end of the 1960s, journalists routinely referred to welfare as a mess, and politicians conducted an agonizing search for the proper means of reforming welfare. In welfare, as in Social Security, therefore, conditions changed from consensus to crisis, although the two programs were out of phase with one another. Social Security's initial crisis coincided with an era of limited acceptance of welfare, although welfare considered as relief or the "dole" never enjoyed widespread acceptance, even in the 1930s. Lorena A. Hickok, a newspaperwoman hired by relief administrator Harry Hopkins to report on the operations of the early New Deal relief programs, advised Hopkins that people in New York City, for example, accepted relief only "as the last resort," having used up their resources, perhaps having been evicted. "There's no food in the house. You've simply got to do something." In the 1950s, with the demand for general assistance down and the demand for social insurance up, both Social Security and welfare were parts of the more general social welfare consensus; in the 1960s, after an initial optimism that welfare recipients could be transformed into workers and integrated into the labor force, welfare became the leading symbol of the welfare state crisis.

As the growing welfare rolls became a federal rather than a state and local problem, a new search began for ways to get the federal government out of the relief business. Where President Roosevelt recommended social insurance, a new generation of reformers, inspired by an optimistic sense that social problems would yield to rational solutions, seized on the idea of rehabilitation. Rehabilitation, an amorphous social process, involved providing people with training, advice, care, or experience in the hope that, once rehabilitated, they would leave the welfare rolls and get a job. John Gardner, President Lyndon B. Johnson's Secretary of Health, Education, and Welfare, described rehabilitation as an all-encompassing philosophy of life that transformed dependent people into independent ones.

By the time Gardner embraced rehabilitation, he could point to impressive success stories, yet nearly all of the stories involved physically disabled persons, not welfare mothers. One story that made the rounds concerned the 1953 case of a sixteen-year-old boy who suffered from a form of paralysis and from double vision. He faced the alternatives of a lifetime of expensive inactivity or, with the right sort of help, a career of productive employment. He had dropped out of high school, further diminishing his chances for a successful career. Then a local counselor discovered him, tested his aptitude, and paid for a course in bookkeeping and typing. Still, his attitude remained poor; he showed "personal maladjustment" and "emotional instability." He needed psychotherapy, and the local vocational rehabilitation agency provided him with this help. Now the newly well-adjusted boy went out and got a job, earning $75 a week as a demonstrator of home furnishings.

The relationship between such case histories and the sort to be found in the AFDC caseload remained unclear; yet, inspired by anecdotes such as the one about the paralyzed boy who took the chip off his shoulder, policymakers recommended rehabilitation as the solution to the welfare "mess."

Rehabilitation, so alien to the spirit of the Social Security Act, gained acceptance as a goal of social policy because of two underlying factors. First, the rising cost of welfare generated demands that something be done to restrain the growth of the programs. Second, changing expectations about who should work and who should stay at home undermined fundamental assumptions about who deserved a pension.

Between Roosevelt's New Deal and Reagan's New Morning, a revolution in labor force expectations occurred. In 1935, policymakers regarded men as natural labor force participants and women as natural child care providers. The entire Social Security apparatus reflected this sexual division of labor. In an explicit sexual reference, for example, the 1939 law referred to workers who died and left behind widows. After 1964, however, female labor force participation rates rose precipitously, and even women caring for young children joined the labor force in large numbers. By 1983, more than half of mothers taking care of children under age 6 expected to work outside of the home. This change, which manpower economist Eli Ginzberg described as "bigger than the atomic bomb or nuclear power," invalidated the fundamental assumption that welfare served a useful social function because it permitted women a dignified alternative to the labor force and strengthened the American family.

Instead, the growth of Social Security, rising costs, and rising rates of female labor participation eroded welfare's legitimacy. As if that were not enough, the substitution of black for white welfare recipients, which also occurred during the troubled 1960s, added to welfare's stigma. Reforming welfare came to mean ending welfare, an impossible task in this country, with its persistent unemployment rate, its pattern of racial discrimination, and its insistence that there be a minimum level of subsistence below which no one, no matter how badly flawed or impaired, should fall. Welfare reform became an exercise in futility, like a dog chasing its tail.

The Benign Era

When Roosevelt proposed the Social Security program in 1935, Congress urged him to raise the level of welfare benefits and to expand the categories eligible for federal financial assistance. In the first fifteen years of the program, Congress continued its pressure on Roosevelt and, after 1945, on Harry Truman as well. Although both presidents' bureaucrats urged that social insurance be given priority over welfare, the politicians scored some impressive victories, such as raising the level of support for old-age assistance (welfare) and establishing Aid to the Blind.

Congress pressed for Aid to the Blind in 1935, and Roosevelt's advisors tried to resist. Although few challenged the right of blind people, charter members of the deserving poor, to operate outside of the conventional patterns of work and retirement, the Roosevelt administration rejected state administered, federally funded pensions on the grounds that the blind had already made an effective appeal to the "sympathies of the public" and did not need special help. Unimpressed with this argument, the Senate took pity on what one congressman described as the "poor blind man with his little tin cup extended." Senator Pat Harrison (D-Miss.), the chairman of the Senate Finance Committee, noted that the sight of several old blind men, who were led into the hearing room by their dogs, "moved" the committee. His committee, reporting to the Senate that only 15 percent of the blind were employed, included welfare grants to the blind in the Social Security legislation. The measure passed the Senate with no opposition, and the House concurred in the conference committee. One congressman, returning from the conference committee, thanked the conferees on "behalf of the thousands of poor blind who must grope their way through a dark world."

Pensions for widows and their dependent children met with even less resistance than Aid to the Blind. Although some southern states, such as Alabama, Georgia, and South Carolina, lacked a program to aid dependent children, most states already ran such a program. In some states, however, these programs suffered from chronic underfunding. In Tennessee, for example, only four percent of the counties availed themselves of the option to participate in 1934, and the state spent only three cents per capita on dependent children. When the federal government initiated Aid to Dependent Children in 1935, no one from Tennessee objected.

Like the other parts of the Social Security Act, Aid to Dependent Children drew on an established agenda of progressive reform. State "mother's pension" programs dated from 1911. The laws, which began in Illinois and Missouri, relied on the logic of deinstitutionalization. If a father died, the reasoning went, a family should be kept together, rather than sending the children off to an orphanage. Theorists maintained that, "a poor home offers a better chance for a child's development than an excellent institution." Mothers' pensions supplied widows with money to keep the family going and functioned as an investment in "home life," "the highest and finest product of civilization," according to the findings of a 1909 White House conference on children and youth. The movement proved so successful that by 1919, thirty-nine states had created mothers' pension laws.

In 1935, officials of the Children's Bureau used the opportunity of the impending Social Security Act to urge that an Aid to Dependent Children program, similar to the state mother's pension laws, be created. The purposes they cited were preventing the "disruption of families on the ground of poverty alone" and allowing a mother to devote herself "to housekeeping and the care of her children." Children's Bureau officials considered and rejected the notion that the widow might work, arguing that unless the widow were highly skilled or a member of a professional group, "her contribution in the home was greater than her earnings outside the home would be."

Economics, it turned out, played a large role in the case for Aid to Dependent Children. Social policy analysts argued, not for the last time, that keeping people at home was cheaper than putting them in institutions. Meanwhile, children in families where the mother tried to be both a homemaker and a wage earner often became "delinquent or seriously neglected" and ended up in orphanages anyway. As Secretary of Labor Frances Perkins noted of mother's pensions, "this has not only proved to be the most satisfactory way from the point of view of the moral, the ethical, and the social principles involved, but it has proved to be vastly the most economical method."

Grace Abbott, the head of the federal Children's Bureau from 1921 to 1934, told Congress the quintessential story about Aid to Dependent Children. It featured a widow with three children. When the father died, they owned a home, but the woman soon found herself unable to make the payments on the mortgage and the bank foreclosed it. In foreclosure, she received $500. She rented a basement apartment and set up a candy and cigar store in the front room; the family were crammed into the back room. Even though the store stayed open all day and late into the night, the widow still found herself short of money. Although her family was inadequately fed and clothed, the mother made only the waiting list when she applied for a state pension, and there she remained for more than two years, running a futile race against destitution. Abbott implied that remedying the widow's situation required only a modest extension of federal power. Congress agreed, and Aid to Dependent Children became federal law.

Although Congress condoned Aid to the Blind and Aid to Dependent Children as reasonable expenditures of public funds, it refused to push federal funds deeper into the traditional welfare system. Like President Roosevelt, the members of Congress respected the difference between a pension and the dole. One politician explained that taxpayers "were perfectly glad" to give welfare to the blind, but refused to assist those whose only claim on welfare was their poverty. The blind, with "a physical handicap that is very distinctive," deserved continuing support; other people, with fewer distinctions, should go get a job. Confided congressional insider Wilbur Mills (D-Ark.) in 1947, while drinking bourbon in House Speaker Sam Rayburn's hideaway office, a program of general assistance to the poor would open a Pandora's box, "a vast system of home relief, a WPA for the Truman depression."

Home relief covered poor people who were neither very old, nor very young, nor blind. At first, the Social Security Act changed nothing about these rag-tag programs, whose financial burden fell on states and, more often than not, on the localities. Even Massachusetts, known for its liberal welfare standards, left the bulk of home relief or general assistance to the towns and cities. A person qualified for aid under the terms of a state law that dated from 1790 and required a person to gain a "legal settlement" by living in a town for five consecutive years.

Other states handled general assistance in ways that reflected local preferences. Pennsylvania coupled general assistance with a work requirement, forcing able-bodied people on welfare to perform labor in projects not in competition with the private sector. In a manner typical of southern states, Tennessee allowed counties to run programs at their discretion. In many mountain counties, grants depended on the benevolence of the local justices of the peace, which was not surprising in a state that, before the Depression, had no state department of public welfare. Administering the general assistance programs, states and localities made the close calls between people expected to work and those excused from the labor force. The federal welfare programs covered those excused from working, leaving only the issue of how generous payments should be. In 1950, on the verge of Social Security's triumph, Congress did not hesitate to create an entirely new welfare category, Aid to the Permanently and Totally Disabled (APTD). At the time, few pointed out that welfare might retard work or that it might be demoralizing. There was little need.

Wartime Reconsideration

At first, the elderly, far more important politically than were dependent children or the blind, gathered the lion's share of federal welfare funds. In 1939, 80 percent of these funds went to the elderly and only 16.9 percent went to dependent children. Eight of the states had still not joined the Aid to Dependent Children program, which helped to account for the fact that nearly three times as many elderly people as dependent children received welfare. Through the war and postwar eras, therefore, welfare policy discussions centered on the elderly, not on welfare mothers and their children.

Already, however, a subtle change affected the way people thought about welfare, the beginning of a shift from a view of welfare as an economic necessity to a sense of welfare as a form of dependency. New Deal reformers, faced with a major depression, had tended to conceive of social problems in economic terms. During the war, behavioral analysis re-emerged as a way of understanding social problems. Although the elderly still received most of the political attention, the psychological analysis applied mainly to children, who represented America's future. During the New Deal, for example, Grace Abbott and other social reformers explained the problems of a widow and her children in terms of a lack of money. The widow required help to pay the rent, buy food, clothe her family. During the war and postwar eras, the woman's situation began to be viewed through a psychological lens. People spoke of the consequences of family break-down and the risks that children might become delinquents. Since a woman could work in the booming wartime economy and bring home a nice paycheck, money no longer appeared to be the pressing issue. Instead, the problem concerned overcoming what one social worker called "emotional shock," and arriving at a "sound basis of mutual understanding and relationship."

In the wartime and postwar economies, the goal of economic security no longer seemed as urgent as did investing in America's future. This new goal focused attention on local attempts to solve social problems, often featuring a search for "healthy" alternatives to welfare. Where the New Deal concentrated on excusing groups from working, the new efforts involved earnest attempts to solicit labor force participation. Where, for example, the New Deal had produced Aid to the Blind, a welfare program, the new style of social welfare featured the work of the President's Committee on the Employment of the Handicapped. Astutely playing on resurgent cultural symbols, the committee, created in 1946, urged the employment of the handi-capped because it was "good business." The blind no longer needed retirement pensions; now the blind could and should participate in the nation's economic revival. In short, optimism and the rhetoric of participation replaced pessimism and the discourse of withdrawal.

In times of prosperity, Americans characteristically have taken an optimistic approach to the solution of social problems, and the post-war era followed the general pattern. For example, Jane Addams, settling in an immigrant neighborhood in Chicago in 1889, started a tradition in which charity workers, who would ultimately become known as social workers, lived among the poor and instructed them in the ways of America. In this manner, social workers helped im-migrants and others to transcend their immediate circumstances and to participate in the larger society. Jane Addams simply assumed that once immigrants learned how to be Americans they would share in America's prosperity. This hands-on, locally oriented, optimistic approach to social policy enjoyed a resurgence in the 1940s.

Social workers welcomed the new emphasis on psychology, be-cause it highlighted their professional skills. Welfare, some social workers complained, robbed social workers of their professional dig-nity and created a public misunderstanding. Welfare programs left little for them to do beyond following rigid rules that had been made by others, and that gave the mistaken impression that only a good nature and good intentions were necessary to become a social worker. "When we are sick we call in a doctor because he has been trained to deal with the ailments of the body," said a spokesman from the Association of Social Workers. Social workers, like doctors, utilized advanced training to diagnose and cure problems. Solving problems of emotional shock, such as those of wartime families broken up by women working and men serving in the military, required just this sort of diagnosis and treatment. Social workers, who had long since given up being ombudsmen for the poor in favor of becoming therapists engaged in individual casework, eagerly offered their help with emotional problems.

In the postwar era, social workers hastened to redefine their public welfare mission in terms of what the Public Welfare Association called the "preventive role of service functions." Such services, by dealing with illness, dependency, and delinquency, helped "individuals and families meet their own problems" and provided social workers with a "maximum degree of administrative flexibility."

The social worker's new public welfare mission suggested a natural division of labor. The Social Security program handled nondiscretionary social welfare by issuing a check. Social workers wanted to become involved in discretionary social welfare, in cases where their intervention might make the difference between adjustment and delinquency, between dignity and dependence. One social worker, for example, spoke of the need to develop, "welfare services or preventive measures that may encourage independence and stimulate self-reliance and self-support."

Not surprisingly, then, Social Security and welfare coexisted peacefully in the period after 1950 when, after the decisive victory of social insurance over welfare, a basic satisfaction with the social welfare system prevailed. Social insurance now carried the bulk of the load, and welfare remained as a residual program that concentrated on worthy members of the deserving poor, such as the blind and the handicapped, or on children facing temporary problems of maladjustment that social workers could cure.

The Problem of Race

This sense of contentment lasted only a short time, and by the late 1950s, conditions had begun to change. The welfare program reached two critical "tipping" points. One concerned the age and nature of welfare recipients and the other involved the race of welfare recipients.

Dependent children and their mothers replaced the elderly as the leading recipients of welfare. In 1957, for the first time, more people received AFDC than received any other category of welfare. Instead of serving widows, AFDC now served mainly families headed by divorced or deserted mothers, for whom the survivors' benefits of Social Security were irrelevant. Right before the passage of the Social Security Act, more than 85 percent of the women on state mother's pension rolls had gotten there because of their husband's death. By mid-1959, fewer than 15 percent of the children on AFDC owed their benefits to the death of their father; most received welfare because their father had left home or never lived there in the first place. By 1962, only 7 percent of the AFDC caseload involved the death of the father, a drop of 30 percent in two decades. This shift has been characterized by Brookings Institution political scientist Gilbert Steiner as "a revolutionary change from the circumstances that brought about the original program."

Even as these changes occurred, welfare generated little controversy, because few people took the growth of the rolls to indicate a welfare crisis. When a family went on welfare, the state was protecting children from poverty. Democrats and Republicans saw the need for such protection and handled welfare policy, in Steiner's phrase, "with few partisan overtones." As late as 1960, after all, the notion that welfare mothers should work had not yet surfaced. America, in the midst of a baby boom, remained a nation of mothers and children, an affluent society that could afford to nurture its young by keeping them at home with their mothers.

If the nation felt it had a welfare problem in 1960, the problem lay in a perception that the family structures of those seeking welfare had deteriorated. More people on welfare implied a growing number of failed marriages and of babies born out of wedlock. It was the absence of the father, not the presence of welfare, that indicated a problem; consequently, social policy sought not so much to curtail welfare payments as to keep families together and prevent mothers from having illegitimate children.

Such trends appeared to confirm the need for welfare services to combat illegitimacy and dependency. Rhode Island congressman Aime Forand expressed the prevailing faith in 1959, after Congress had already started a small program of subsidized welfare services, noting that welfare recipients were people with "special needs requiring knowledgeable service for their solution."

The service approach differed sharply from failing to serve needy children, as Louisiana officials discovered in 1960. Governor Jimmie Davis pledged to cut off welfare payments to women and children who lived in "unsuitable homes." The governor invoked newly passed state legislation that denied welfare to a woman who bore an illegitimate child after she had already received a welfare check or who cohabited with a man "without benefit of formal marriage." In July, the governor cut 22,501 children from the state's welfare rolls.

When Secretary of Health, Education, and Welfare Arthur Flemming heard of the governor's action, he immediately sought the counsel of the department's lawyers. On January 17, 1961, three days before John F. Kennedy's inauguration, Flemming ruled that states could not impose a plan that denied aid to a child in an unsuitable home, if the child remained in the home. States, in other words, could not punish children because they were illegitimate or because their mothers lived with a man without marrying him. In effect, Flemming decided that Louisiana's law, but not the practice of paying welfare to illegitimate children, was unsuitable. When Abraham Ribicoff, Kennedy's appointee as Secretary of Health, Education, and Welfare, took over from Flemming on January 20, he concurred in Flemming's ruling.

In particular, Louisiana offended federal authorities because it had introduced the divisive matter of race into discussions of welfare. Although no one dwelled on the fact, only 5 percent of the Louisianan children found to be in "unsuitable" homes were white. Louisiana's governor wanted to turn welfare into a racial issue at a time when civil rights, particularly in the South, was fast emerging as the nation's major domestic concern.

The association between welfare and race appeared natural, if one considered the disproportionate number of poor people who were black and the fact that Social Security coverage came most slowly to occupations, such as farm labor and domestic service, in which many blacks were employed. Despite this natural association, the federal welfare programs—aid to the elderly, the blind, and dependent children—began as benefits reserved nearly exclusively for whites. In 1939, for example, 86 percent of the ADC caseload consisted of white children.

As the Louisiana incident revealed, the presence of blacks on welfare rolls generated political controversy in the South, where the bulk of the black population still lived in the 1930s and 1940s. Southern congressmen, who had accrued considerable seniority and power, protected local prerogatives to determine who should receive welfare and resisted national standards for welfare benefits. Leaders of black organizations, such as the National Association for the Advancement of Colored People (NAACP), made little headway with these congressmen when they tried, for example, to gain Social Security coverage for domestic workers. In 1949, Congressman "Muley" Doughton of North Carolina belittled Clarence Mitchell of the NAACP for suggesting that domestics be covered. The congressman asked Mitchell to tell him about reliable women willing to work as servants for $9 a week, "If so, I wish you would give us their names. I can think I could find a lot of people who would like to employ them." In such an atmosphere, discussions of race tended to be muted.

Just as southerners saw no need to bring up race, so social workers downplayed the connection between race and welfare. An official HEW pamphlet, issued in the early 1960s, describing the AFDC program as a means "to help needy families find strength, security, and hope," contained two illustrations of groups of welfare recipients. Neither included a single black person. The demographic breakdown featured in the pamphlet said nothing about race; instead, it noted that AFDC "is needed more often in the cities." Social workers, accustomed to working with Jews and Italians in urban settings, still thought of blacks as the new ethnic group living in the old neighborhood.

Then, in 1961, as the newly elected Kennedy administration considered what, if anything, to do about welfare, an event occurred that challenged the liberal assumptions about welfare and brought race into the open as a subject of public discussion. The event acquired a symbolic importance that far outstripped its practical influence over the level of welfare payments. It became known as the battle of Newburgh.

Newburgh, a mildly depressed town on the west bank of the Hudson River, not far from the rich baronies of the Hudson Valley elite, such as the Roosevelts of Hyde Park, contained a declining labor force engaged in making pocket books, working in other garment trades, or who commuted elsewhere. The demographic trends in Newburgh traced a familiar pattern. After 1950, Newburgh's population underwent a gentle decline, almost exclusively among whites. As more than 5,000 blacks moved into Newburgh, a greater number of whites left. In 1957, for the first time, more blacks than whites received AFDC in the city of Newburgh. By 1960, furthermore, the ratio of taxpayers to welfare recipients reached an all-time low, a source of considerable concern. Paying welfare to about one in twenty of Newburgh's residents cost the city more than did police protection.

A small city of 31,000 people, Newburgh operated in an informal manner, delegating most of its administrative operations to a city manager. In October 1960, the city council selected Joseph McDowell Mitchell as the city manager, and he made welfare an area of special concern. In the spring of 1961, Mitchell devised a means to separate those who deserved welfare from those whom he regarded as chiselers. He issued an edict that all heads of households on welfare had to come to the police station to pick up their checks. A parade of elderly and infirm peopled marched to the station, where they participated in what former military man Mitchell referred to as a "muster." People with canes and women with babies all suffered the indignity of reporting to the police station.

Mitchell, it became clear, wanted to treat the receipt of welfare as a crime. In so doing, he played upon potent images of the era. Mitchell's treatment of welfare recipients in Newburgh resembled the treatment of freedom riders, making their way through the South to challenge the segregation laws, received from Alabaman politicians. In both cases, white leaders sought to gain favor with white voters by challenging the legitimacy of newly acquired black civil rights.

Instead of hiding from the association between race and welfare, as the social workers and southern congressmen did, Mitchell reveled in it. He quickly issued a report on welfare in which the references to blacks were so thinly veiled as almost to be highlighted. The report blamed Newburgh's welfare problem on a "steady influx of outsiders principally from Southern states . . . who apparently have no desire to take root and become part of community life." Mitchell feared these blacks would become permanent outsiders, chronic welfare recipients, constant drains on the city's budget. Unlike the city's Jewish population, which had, for example, yielded the city's most prominent lawyer, the new arrivals offered nothing, he thought. Mitchell made it clear that he did not wish to engage in rehabilitation; he preferred to close the city to new black arrivals. He advocated that any newcomer to the city (read black person) be required to demonstrate that he or she had come to Newburgh with a job offer in hand before that person could receive welfare.

Mitchell, now being watched by the national press, presented the city with a new set of welfare rules in June 1961. Following the lead of Louisiana, Mitchell urged that Newburgh welfare recipients who had another illegitimate child be thrown off the rolls. Invoking his own version of the suitable home requirement, he asked local welfare workers to investigate the "home environment" of each welfare applicant. If the home were determined not to be satisfactory, then the child should be placed in foster care.

At base, Mitchell wanted a return to the traditional poor law, with its notions that each community should take care of its own poor on its own terms. Mitchell defined the Newburgh community as the one that had existed before 1950. He therefore sought to deny blacks permanent settlement in the town on the theory that they represented a social liability; they would ultimately appear on the city's ledgers as debits rather than as property owners and hence credits. He also put restrictions on the receipt of welfare, such as a provision denying welfare to anyone who refused a job and one allowing welfare to be paid in vouchers good only for food, rather than in cash that could be used for luxuries or alcohol.

Mitchell's plan sparked a national debate, one of the nation's first on the subject of welfare reform. Politicians supported Mitchell to the degree that it suited their purposes. Barry Goldwater, a prophet of the conservative movement and a contender for the Republican presidential nomination, chose to single out Mitchell for special praise, even as Nelson Rockefeller, New York's liberal Republican governor and a rival of Goldwater's for the 1964 nomination, decided to put legal roadblocks in Mitchell's way. After Goldwater met with Mitchell, he described the meeting as "one American's admiration for [the efforts of] another to protect my taxes." Goldwater said that he was tired of "chiselers," who had no intention of working, being on welfare.

Liberals reacted with alarm. Mitchell wanted to set back the clock to an age in which blacks lived segregated lives in the American South. He demanded a form of ideological purity in an age that the liberals considered to be beyond ideology. He believed that enough jobs existed for everyone, at a time when modern technology left many unskilled workers unable to compete. Mitchell's plan, in short, reflected the shortcomings of a man who lacked the mental agility to comprehend the realities of modern American life. Mitchell's ideas, declared the *New York Times*, were "simplistic," his arguments ones that permitted "a clear differentiation between good guys and bad guys." Liberal journalists portrayed Mitchell as a dangerous anti-intellectual who appointed a physical education teacher as the city's welfare commissioner and referred to college-educated welfare workers as "brainwashed social beatniks."

Social workers felt that, above all, the Newburgh situation was a test of society's faith in professionals. In their view, Mitchell's major mistake was wanting to downgrade, rather than upgrade, professional service. Leaders of the social work community pointed out that most public assistance workers lacked a college education and fewer than 20 percent had training in social work. Such workers, although "eager for more training," determined eligibility for assistance in a "superficial" way and lacked the skills to provide the counseling that made people "independent and self-supporting." Complicated personal problems required "the expert assistance of trained social workers." To think otherwise violated the era's faith in the ability of experts to solve complicated problems. It resembled, they said, replacing "atomic engineers" with "tenth graders to build missiles," or asking "auto mechanics . . . to practice medicine."

Energized by the Newburgh crisis, John F. Kennedy became the first American president since Roosevelt to make welfare a domestic priority. He realized that Newburgh's situation framed a clear policy choice. On the right, Mitchell and his national supporters wanted to limit the growth of the welfare rolls by restricting welfare to the "truly needy" and limiting the generosity of welfare grants. On the left, social workers and their liberal supporters hoped to contain the rolls by rehabilitating welfare beneficiaries and producing, in the words of a *New York Times* reporter, "the regeneration of the will-to-work and the ability-to-work of the needy." Civil rights formed the subtext of this choice. Those on the right, who saw black migration to the North as disruptive to the fabric of society, regarded welfare reform as a means of stemming the rapid pace of social change. Those on the left, who viewed black migration as an inevitable feature of modern life, considered welfare reform as a means of reaching the goal of integration, as a source of opportunity.

President Kennedy sided with the liberals and took steps to advance their agenda for welfare reform, although the president viewed the entire matter in highly tempered and pragmatic terms. Politics, in this area of domestic policy as in so many others, dictated prudence, if only to maintain the good will of the southerners who dominated Congress. The changes of the Kennedy era took on a permissive cast that permitted the states wide latitude in implementing the rehabilitation approach. Whenever possible, Kennedy, appealing to a higher social good, beyond the immediate southern concern with civil rights legislation, related welfare reform to his efforts to get the economy "moving again" and to win the Cold War.

Early in his administration, Kennedy sent social welfare measures to Congress and asked for quick action, to stem the threat of a recession. He included a proposal to grant states temporary authority to pay welfare to families with unemployed fathers. This proposal matched one he had made in 1958 as a Massachusetts senator and also reflected the recommendations of the Advisory Council on Public Assistance that reported in January 1960 and of a transition task force headed by Wilbur J. Cohen, a former assistant to Arthur Altmeyer and now the Assistant Secretary for Legislation at the Department of Health, Education, and Welfare (HEW). When HEW Secretary Abraham Ribicoff met with the Committee on Ways and Means in February 1961, he promised to have a more complete welfare reform plan ready by the next session of Congress. Ribicoff, even more than Kennedy, regarded welfare as an important priority because of the time he had devoted to it as governor of Connecticut in the 1950s.

Ribicoff encouraged social work organizations such as the National

Social Welfare Assembly, government experts such as Cohen, and others interested in welfare to produce a coherent series of legislative recommendations that embodied the rehabilitation approach. Of the various internal and external reports submitted, the one by the Ad Hoc Committee on Public Welfare attracted the most attention. Ribicoff met personally with this group on September 8, 1961.

When the group assembled in his office, Ribicoff picked up a copy of *US News and World Report* that featured a story entitled "The Growing Scandal in Relief." The article quoted such anecdotes as the one about a woman with 23 children, 15 of whom were illegitimate, who received nearly $1,000 a month in welfare benefits. "You are dealing with sensation," said Ribicoff, who mentioned that NBC News and *Look* magazine wanted to interview him on the subject of welfare. Then, warming to his task, Ribicoff told the group that he wanted "to accentuate the positive," perhaps by renaming the Bureau of Public Assistance, the Bureau of Family Rehabilitation. When a member of the group told him, "our strongest recommendation is a stepped up program of rehabilitation service to the ADC families by trained personnel," the secretary showed considerable interest. "If you are able to remove people from the relief rolls and take a positive approach, you are going to find someone who really believes in this in Congress," said Ribicoff, noting that, all too often, "people feel uncomfortable with slum people and salve their conscience by blaming those who work with them." Ribicoff congratulated the group on its efforts and asked for positive stories about welfare he could use in speeches, to counteract the sensational stories appearing in the popular press.

Members of the social work establishment responded enthusiastically to the secretary's request and kept Assistant Secretary Cohen supplied with a steady stream of upbeat welfare stories. From Colorado came a clipping from a local newspaper headed "Trujillo Passes Air Academy Exams," with an inked notation that Trujillo, "an outstanding student," grew up on welfare. Another clipping featured a picture, like a wedding portrait, of Miss Codie Ridgeway, a senior at the Asbury Hospital School in Salinas Kansas who, the story noted, had won the "Miss Methodist Student Nurse" award. Ridgeway, explained the director of the Yuma County (Colorado) Department of Public Welfare, received ADC throughout high school.

Ellen Winston, an influential state welfare director from North Carolina, sent Cohen a series of case studies that also illustrated the potential of welfare recipients for meaningful social participation. The families in these cases often had met with an unfortunate occurrence, such as sickness, and many contained exceptionally gifted individuals. Welfare had invariably been the agent that had preserved the family and enabled the gifted individuals, nearly always children, to realize their potential and achieve their ambitions. Viewed from this perspective, welfare prevented poverty in the short run and augmented the nation's wealth in the long run. For example, Peggy's father was "physically incapacitated" and could not "hold regular employment." The father received welfare, which proved of great value to Peggy, who had a "high IQ." Peggy, continued Winston, "is capable of doing much more advanced work than her classmates and her teacher has given her additional work because of this. This family is doing everything they can to help themselves and take great pride in Peggy and her accomplishments." The stories portrayed welfare as an institution from which talented people graduated and matriculated to the wider world, much as a young math prodigy might pass through the Bronx School of Science on his way to MIT.

Even the cheerful stories contained some sobering sides, as the social workers unabashedly subjected their clients to intrusive regimens of self-help. The story of Alice, intended as positive evidence of the rehabilitation approach, illustrated the paces through which social workers put their charges. Born a "spastic," Alice grew up wearing braces on her feet and legs. Her mother had died when Alice was young, and her father led "a rather worthless life," because, revealingly, of a "lack of skilled training." The father eventually sent Alice to live with an aunt, who secured welfare for Alice and obtained treatment at an orthopedic hospital. Alice began to attend school, and despite Alice's poor grades, her social worker spotted her "excellent progress in social adjustment." Indeed, the social worker, perceptive in the extreme, noticed that Alice, "plain in appearance and physically handicapped, had a burning desire to be a beautician" and "through skilled caseworker services" helped Alice "to realize this ambition." Still, Alice needed more work, in the form of psychiatric treatment, which "helped Alice to resolve some of her deep-seated and mixed-up emotions." All of this intensive therapy paid off when, on her eighteenth birthday, just as her welfare grant expired, she "completed her course in beauty culture,. . . received her certificate," and emerged "employed and able to support herself, despite her handicap."

These stories of welfare as a engine of opportunity served to rebut the horror stories featured in *US News and World Report* and to shape a more positive image for welfare. In this regard, they, along with the report of the Ad Hoc Committee on Public Welfare, which stressed the need for rehabilitative services to help families become self-supporting and independent, laid the groundwork for Ribicoff's welfare reform proposals.

In December 1961, Ribicoff announced his desire to update the welfare program. "The byword of our new program is prevention—and where it is too late—rehabilitation, a fresh start," he said. His formal proposals combined stricter enforcement, such as renewed efforts to locate deserting fathers and combat welfare fraud, and rehabilitation services. "If we are going to avoid as far as possible more illegitimate births, if we are going to help these families become responsible citizens," wrote Ribicoff, "we have to render to this category of family special services that we have seen can be effective." He mentioned placing problem families in small caseloads, making sure trained social workers saw problem families, increasing the frequency of home visits, and removing children from hazardous home situations.

President Kennedy chose to make the new public welfare proposals a centerpiece of his domestic legislation for 1962. Welfare reform, although crossed with the conundrums of race, still generated less controversy than national health insurance or measures more directly related to civil rights. In February, Kennedy sent Congress an unprecedented special message devoted to public welfare, in which he described his program, uniting the two polarities of liberal thought, as tough and compassionate. "We have here," the president declared, "a realistic program which will pay dividends on every dollar invested. It can move some persons off the assistance rolls entirely, enable others to attain a higher degree of self-confidence and independence, encourage children to grow strong in mind and body, train welfare workers in the skills which will help make these achievements possible and simplify and improve welfare administration."

Social workers hastened to bless the new legislation. They welcomed the emphasis on individual aid and service, described by a spokesman for the National Social Welfare Assembly as a "more intensive investment in social service in order to help them find the means to self-support or a more satisfactory way of life." Elizabeth Wickenden, a veteran observer of the social work scene with considerable influence in Washington, commended Ribicoff for seeking the views of so many in the social work establishment. Speaking before the Senate Finance Committee, she said that the entire effort to turn public assistance around depended on increasing the number of professionally qualified social workers in public welfare agencies.

Congress quickly approved the plan. In essence, the 1962 law allowed the federal government to match state funds for staff training and rehabilitative services at the rate of three federal dollars for every state dollar contributed. In addition, the law made the 1961 temporary extension of the AFDC program to cover unemployed parents permanent, authorized federal grants for state community work and training programs, and gave the secretary of health, education, and welfare the authority to spend money for social work training, fellowships, and special short courses of study.

Despite the groundswell of support for the legislation, Ribicoff's assurances that services "can be effective," and Kennedy's declarations that the program would pay dividends, the new approach rested on the thinnest of evidence. Little more than a veneer of hopeful anecdotes, limited demonstration projects, and professional self-confidence supported the 1962 public welfare amendments. No one really knew if significant numbers of welfare recipients could be rehabilitated. In the postwar era, the idea became an article of faith among the interlocking groups of experts who advised the Kennedy administration.

Indeed, these advisors willfully ignored much of the evidence available to them, an example of which was a survey of settlement house workers conducted by the National Federation of Settlements and Neighborhood Centers. This survey reported the negative image of relief clients in Cleveland who were subjected to "daily insults," could find no one to cash their checks, and who received "brusque treatment" from doctors. Could rehabilitation succeed in the face of this negative image? In Boston, the survey noted, welfare recipients went to work without telling their social workers, "distorting the values and attitudes" of their children, "who are fully aware of the mother's activity." Could rehabilitation reduce the incentives for breaking the welfare rules? The survey also revealed new types of welfare recipients in Tacoma, Washington, for example, who had "little regard for neighborhood standards," who "misused the funds," who "neglected their children," and who "openly flouted their prostitution." "At this point," a Tacoma welfare worker reported, "our 'good ADC mothers' are taking a terrific beating as a group for the sins of the poor ones. But more serious is the slackness of the poor ADC mother, the abuse of the children, and the growing contempt that the neighborhood and the community at large is exhibiting to all ADC mothers and to social workers." Were rehabilitation services a match for all that?

Such problems to the contrary, passage of the law meant that the social welfare system that had been dominated by social insurance would now be given a decisive rehabilitation twist. Taken together, rehabilitation and social insurance constituted a positive approach to social welfare, one that, in 1962, helped to quell the growing controversy over welfare and promised much future success.

Wars on Poverty

Although the social workers hedged nearly all of their claims with qualifications, the passage of the 1962 amendments created a series of expectations. Now that the states had the authority to rehabilitate welfare beneficiaries, policymakers expected the growth of the AFDC rolls to halt, particularly given the booming economy of the era. Taking over after the assassination of John F. Kennedy in November 1963, President Lyndon B. Johnson added to the expectations by declaring war on poverty. When welfare recipients continued to grow in number despite all of the apparent attention being paid to them, welfare entered a state of crisis that required still another new sort of response.

The idea of a war on poverty reflected the optimism of the postwar era far more than it did the New Deal conditions from which welfare and Social Security had arisen. Lyndon Johnson rallied the nation to the goal of ending poverty; Franklin Roosevelt, faced with the ravages of the Depression, urged the nation toward the much more modest goal of economic recovery. When President Johnson delivered his first State of the Union address in January 1964 and announced, "This administration today, here and now, declares unconditional war on poverty in America," he sounded less like Roosevelt than like Herbert Hoover, who had inaugurated his administration by saying, "we shall soon with the help of God be in sight of the day when poverty shall be banished from this land."

Johnson plunged right into the war on poverty, hoping to extend the New Deal legacy he had inherited from Roosevelt and confident, too, that the war on poverty could become his program, rather than something that reflected his political stewardship of Kennedy's proposals. The day after the assassination he summoned Walter Heller, the Minnesota economist who chaired the Council of Economic Advisers, and told him to proceed with the anti-poverty program.

Kennedy had set his Council of Economic Advisers to work on the program early in 1963. Worrying, as always, about his image, President Kennedy wanted to balance his proposed tax cut, which promised to bring the middle class and the rich substantial gains, with a proposal for a poverty program, which offered help to the people in urban ghettos and rural hollows for whom tax breaks were distant dreams.

Kennedy's situation resembled President Roosevelt's in 1934. He wanted to take a decisive action that would demonstrate presidential leadership; he hoped to lead public opinion in a manner that would show foresight rather than rash judgment. Little grass-roots demand preceded the War on Poverty, and even less support emerged for the specific anti-poverty measures that Kennedy initiated, and Johnson saw passed into law.

As with the Social Security Act, Johnson's War on Poverty reflected the ideas of a specific set of experts, rather than the desires of the public. And as in the case of Social Security, a compliant Congress, faced with extraordinary circumstances, allowed the president a great deal of control over both the items on the policy agenda and the approaches taken toward them.

Although the problem of poverty differed from the problem of economic security, Kennedy's and Roosevelt's advisors shared a common intellectual outlook. Each president's team of advisors, despite the years that separated them, condemned the ill effects of politics on social policy. Each wanted to substitute what they perceived as impartial expertise for the pork barrel behavior of local politicians. The New Deal experts, struck by the inadequacy and inefficiency of local relief efforts, favored vesting more power in the national government and creating national social insurance programs; the Kennedy advisors — economists, sociologists, and psychologists who were products of the postwar resurgence in local self-help efforts — struck by the apparent failure even of the New Deal programs to promote economic opportunity, particularly among blacks, favored establishing a new bureaucratic structure, with direct links to federal experts, and initiating rehabilitation efforts.

While he was influenced by these experts, President Kennedy nonetheless relied heavily on advice from members of his family. Early in the administration, Robert Kennedy, the attorney general, and Eunice Kennedy Shriver, a former employee of President Truman's Committee on the Prevention and Control of Delinquency, grew interested in the problems of juvenile delinquency. When the poverty program came under discussion, Robert Kennedy brought ideas and experts from his juvenile delinquency endeavors to the president's attention. In particular, he advanced the notion of "community action." Community action eventually became an important feature of Lyndon Johnson's full-scale war on poverty. Johnson, as if to close the loop, selected Eunice Shriver's husband to run the Office of Economic Opportunity, the command post for the war.

The exact meaning of *community action* remained vague right up to the point when President Johnson signed the Economic Opportunity Act into law on August 20, 1964. Modeled after Robert Kennedy's delinquency projects, community action agencies provided a means, according to Michael Katz, of "shaking the system and forcing change on reluctant school administrators, welfare and employment service officials, and even settlement houses and Community Chest leaders." The law described community action projects as antipoverty efforts that developed employment opportunities, improved human performance, motivation, and productivity, or bettered the conditions under which people lived, learned and worked. To complete such projects, the act directed local communities to designate public or private non-profit agencies as grant recipients. These agencies, expected to mount a comprehensive attack on poverty, faced the task of converting the institutional chaos of streams of money entering the community from all levels of government into a coherent, smoothly running program that lifted the poor out of poverty and helped them stay out.

As in any rehabilitation effort, specific models, rather than the vaguely worded guidelines, served as the basis for action. The War on Poverty drew on earlier projects, funded first by private foundations, as in the Ford Foundation's Gray Areas project, and then by federal agencies, that tried to control problems of urban poverty and of juvenile delinquency. These projects relied on psychological theories as a means of explaining social problems and suggesting possible solutions. The projects proceeded from the assumption that poverty reflected more than a lack of money. In the words of a 1963 prospectus from a Ford Foundation project, poverty resulted from, "inadequate education, low or non-existent income, limited job opportunities, dilapidated and overcrowded housing, poor physical and mental health, an inclination toward delinquency and crime," all, "interacting in a manner which renders it virtually impossible for the disadvantaged child, adult, or family to break out of the cycle of poverty."

Experts in the 1960s faced the same dilemma as did the creators of social insurance. Although they realized they could simply give people money, they saw the limitations of this approach, since it alleviated but did not solve the problem. Maintaining people's income at government expense promised to be a never-ending process and to create an insupportable future financial burden. Instead of dependency, the poverty warriors hoped to develop self-sufficiency among the poor and in this manner to eliminate poverty. Cash grants, whatever their immediate effects, defeated that goal. In a similar manner, Social Security's creators came to view welfare as a crushing burden and turned instead to self-help in the form of social insurance.

In the case of the poverty planners, self-help meant rehabilitation, which, in their optimistic way, they saw as a means of eliminating poverty, not just controlling it. That implied a coordinated attack on all of the causes of poverty, and that brought the poverty planners to the notion of community action.

Unlike the creators of social insurance, the poverty planners contended with the confounding problems of race relations. Self-help, according to the psychological rubric from which the planners drew, depended on the development of self-confidence at both the individual and the community level. Ghetto residents needed to feel a sense of their own power and ability if they were to realize the possibilities of helping themselves and rising above poverty. Blacks would have to gain confidence in their communities, and ultimately in their race, in order to overcome the feeling that, in the words of a Harlem teenager, "I can't solve my problem unless I attempt to solve it with a white person at my side." At the same time, the local community action projects depended on white experts for advice and for medical, educational, and other services. The War on Poverty consequently relied on reconciling elite and grass-roots approaches to social policy at a time of deepening distrust between whites and blacks. Almost as soon as the Community Action program went into operation, for example, race riots broke out in the nation's cities, including a 1965 riot in the Watts section of Los Angeles that marked the end of the nonviolent, integrationist phase of the civil rights movement.

Like the public welfare amendments of 1962, the War on Poverty relied on untested theory for its design and unrestrained enthusiasm for its implementation. Rehabilitation proved so irresistible, so appropriate for the times, that the results of earlier experiments appeared not to matter. Often, the earlier projects, such as Community Progress Incorporated (CPI) in New Haven, Connecticut, practiced conventional social work of a type difficult to distinguish from the actions of caseworkers in regular welfare programs, as a 1964 CPI case record indicated.

The case concerned BJ and his family, who had moved to New Haven from the South in 1955. BJ's education "took place as much in the cotton fields as it did in school." A bad student, he earned the label "incorrigible fighter" and dropped out of school in ninth grade. The case record showed that CPI made contact with BJ through a neighborhood employment worker who was "a Negro and a lifelong resident of the young man's neighborhood." In time, caseworkers for the project managed to provide BJ with a job as a stock boy and elevator operator in a downtown store. "We know that BJ is still a high-risk placement but we hope with our continued support it will be a successful one," the record concluded. The case bore a resemblance to that of Alice, the spastic who became a beautician; in each case, social welfare professionals helped their client overcome handicaps that created emotional disturbances and blocked their vocational progress. Alice overcame her physical handicap and became a hairdresser, BJ surmounted his racial handicap and became a stock boy. Whether similar labor-intensive, intrusive methods would work on a national scale never became clear.

Nor did authorities delve too deeply into the work training programs that preceded the War on Poverty. Begun with grandiose hopes of endowing ghetto residents with valuable skills, the earlier programs had degenerated into simple exercises in discipline. Started as training programs, they became what might be described as "pre-training" programs stressing such things, according to sociologists Peter Marris and Martin Rein, as "regularity, punctuality, neatness, how to approach a prospective employer, how to handle the conflicts and frustrations of work relationships, how to tolerate others and respect the legitimate expectations of a boss." The links between acquiring these attributes and finding a job, holding a job, and rising above poverty never became clear.

Community action formed one flank of the War on Poverty, and more traditional job training, health care, and educational programs formed another. Consequently, although the War on Poverty reflected the frustration of Kennedy and Johnson administration officials who perceived a lack of creativity in public welfare programs, it nonetheless bore a close resemblance to the 1962 amendments recommended by the social work establishment: both programs depended on massive infusions of services and education to cure poverty and welfare dependency. A 1963 report prepared by the Social Security Administration, "Unmet Need in a Land of Abundance," set the tone. "Although services cannot substitute for income," the report stated, "certain types of service might counteract some of the effects of poverty and thus help to break the cycle of cultural deprivation that is often associated with poverty."

Unlike other rehabilitation efforts contemplated at the time, however, the War on Poverty sought to change not only the residents of ghettos but the ghettos themselves: it was a salvage operation aimed at places as well as people, a blend of urban renewal and self-help.

Because the War on Poverty received such attention from President Johnson, who announced its goals in such bold, uncompromising terms, it added to the general expectations about reducing the welfare rolls. Ending poverty would mean rehabilitating the poor and re-

---

Welfare's State, 1935–1967

ducing the welfare rate, a simple test of the complex theories that produced the 1962 amendments and 1964 war on poverty legislation.

Simply put, the programs failed the test. It does not take regression analysis to determine the rising welfare rate. From 3.1 million people on AFDC in 1960, the number rose to 4.3 million in 1965, and 6.7 million in 1969. Meanwhile, the percentage of non-whites on AFDC grew steadily, from 32 percent in 1950 to 46 percent in 1967. In Milwaukee, for example, by 1965 most of the people on welfare were black.

Making matters worse, evidence soon arrived that showed incompetence in the local management of welfare programs, despite the new legislation. The most celebrated case concerned the District of Columbia. Senator Robert Byrd (D-W.Va.) asked the nonpartisan General Accounting Office to investigate the welfare caseload in that city and determine how many people receiving welfare met the terms of the law. The GAO selected a sample of 236 AFDC cases and found 60 percent of the families in the sample to be ineligible. Common violations involved the presence of a man in the house, higher income than reported to authorities, and mothers working without telling authorities or reporting the income. The GAO report included juicy vignettes of the more flagrant cases, such as that of a 24-year-old mother of four children, fathered by three different men. The mother never informed the local social worker of the fourth child's birth. Deciding to investigate for themselves, the authorities conducted an early morning "raid" on the mother's home one Sunday and found the father of the two youngest children, who admitted to spending the night and being employed, hiding in the bathroom.

Defenders of the rehabilitation approach reacted ambivalently to such revelations by those who wished to discredit public assistance programs. On the one hand, the social workers deplored fraud; on the other hand, they questioned the legitimacy of a system that permitted midnight raids, forced women to choose between honesty and subsistence, and required welfare recipients to uphold higher standards of virtue than the general public. Similarly, the social workers regarded the rise in the welfare rolls as a reflection of the slow pace of implementing the 1962 law, realistic coping methods on the part of the poor, and the decline of anachronistic and repressive practices that had kept the rolls at artificially low levels in the past.

In the case of Washington, D.C., all of these factors came into play. Administrative incompetence and fraud, abetted by the relaxation of anachronistic rules, such as the one barring illicit sex, accounted for rising welfare rolls, but so too did the fact that the city stood in what Elizabeth Wickenden called the "direct path" of black northern migration. "Since many of these are relative newcomers—unskilled, undereducated, and poorly adjusted to modern urban life—they are especially vulnerable to all the factors that make for [welfare] dependency," Wickenden noted.

As Wickenden and others pointed out, the service strategy in Washington, D.C. and elsewhere took hold slowly or not at all. The permissive legislation did not require a state to pay welfare to a family with an unemployed father and a homemaker mother, and half chose not to do so. Furthermore, many states never mounted a serious rehabilitation effort but instead learned how to rig the system. If a state agreed to provide such vague things as, in the case of Wisconsin, "counseling regarding environmental conditions seriously contributing to illegitimacy" and then designated a particular case as a "defined service case," it received special federal funds to pay the caseworker's salary. Increased federal funds authorized by the 1962 amendments often went to social workers, not welfare recipients.

For all that the failure of the service approach to stop the rise in welfare concerned matters of scale and execution, it also reflected confusions and contradictions imbedded within the approach itself. Updating the welfare laws, as Ribicoff proposed to do, meant ending anachronistic practices, such as the "man in the house" rules, that had served to limit the size of the rolls in the past. All other things being equal, modernizing the laws implied expanding the welfare rolls. Rehabilitation, in the form of welfare services and community action, constituted an unclear response to these rising welfare rolls. Few knew, for example, exactly how to change the environmental conditions that produced illegitimacy, yet federal authorities urged local governments, such as the ones in Wisconsin, to do so. The lack of clarity in the notion of "helping to plan a mother and child's future" also hindered local implementation efforts. Flexibility and discretion, the very things social workers and poverty warriors had worked so hard to obtain, also proved to be very unstable concepts on which to base the work of a large and growing bureaucracy.

Some services funded as part of the War on Poverty fueled the resentment of the white establishment and created a backlash that undermined the already thin support for the program. It was one thing to encourage black self-expression and quite another, as historian Allen Matusow notes, to fund the Black Arts Theatre's production of LeRoi Jones's *Jello*—in which Jack Benny's valet, Rochester, rises up and kills his white oppressors. It was one thing to encourage a community's self-confidence and quite another to pay organizers who trained people in techniques to harass the city government. It was one thing to redirect the flow of resources toward a particular community and quite another to use the War on Poverty as a means of increasing the number of community residents on welfare.

Legal services, an important feature of both the War on Poverty and the service strategy, exemplified the confusions and contradictions of the approach. One reason that ghetto residents lacked self-confidence or "community competence" was that they felt that the legal system was rigged against them: it was expensive, intrusive, and threatening. One solution was to provide ghetto residents with a free source of legal advice that would make them the equals of opposing parties—with deeper pockets—in the courts. Soon, however, it appeared that the legal services demanded by ghetto residents were conflicting with the larger, rehabilitation-oriented goals imposed from outside the ghetto. Planners wanted strong families; ghetto residents used legal services to obtain divorces. Planners wanted to end welfare dependency; ghetto residents used legal services to challenge capricious denials of welfare grants. Contesting the decisions of the welfare department became an important part of the Legal Aid process. Legal Aid lawyers exploited whatever part of the law might provide a means for their particular clients to get welfare and took it upon themselves to fight such practices as length-of-residence requirements and man in the house rules. As one lawyer said in 1965, his role was not to act as "mere technician" but "to utilize the legal system to help change the very nature of the welfare system." He was talking about making the system more permissive, not more oriented toward rehabilitation. In so doing, he and his fellow Legal Aid lawyers created an overt conflict between the advertised goals of reducing dependence on welfare and those of building power and self-confidence.

These various sources of vagueness and confusion led not to a reduction in the welfare rolls but rather its opposite—a significant increase in what authorities called the welfare "take-up" rate. By 1971, an estimated 90 percent of those eligible for welfare received it. In the past, this rate had been much lower, perhaps 33 percent in the early 1960s. The increase meant that the tangible result of the service initiatives of the decade had been an increase in welfare rates and welfare expenditures, a direct contradiction of the promises made to legislators.

Coached by the community action program, welfare beneficiaries pressed for larger grants. During the 1960s, welfare recipients, bringing the social worker's language about a culture of poverty down to street level, came to see themselves as victims of an unjust and inhumane society, even though, paradoxically, they accepted the hospitality of this unjust society in the form of welfare. Hence, public housing programs required expansion, argued a black leader in 1966, because black people suffered from the "ravages of a punitive, prejudiced society." Viewing the problem that way, welfare recipients followed the model of the civil rights movement and organized to secure their rights, in this case the right to welfare.

George Wiley, an articulate spokesman with experience in the civil rights movement, founded the National Welfare Rights Organization (NWRO) in the middle 1960s. Although it represented a tiny fraction of welfare recipients, it acquired an instant legitimacy because it represented the only group of welfare beneficiaries whose views could easily be solicited. Soon the testimony of the NWRO became a feature of congressional hearings on welfare.

Conditions were now ripe for a white backlash. Having engaged in an idealistic effort to end poverty and rehabilitate ghetto residents, the nation now found itself abused, tormented, and threatened by the very people it had sought to help. Whites resented the ingratitude of blacks yet felt a sense of guilt that blacks remained so far below them on the economic ladder. Blacks blamed whites for not making greater efforts at rehabilitation and felt a sense of frustration, and of inferiority, for not accomplishing more in such an apparently wealthy society. Since the results of the rehabilitation effort appeared to satisfy no one, the consensus that produced the 1962 welfare amendments and the 1964 War on Poverty soon fell apart. Politicians, who had once treated welfare as a good government measure that required bipartisan cooperation, began to rethink their commitments.

Congress soon reacted to the changing mores and insisted on a return to "basic values." In 1967, a year marked by urban riots even as welfare rates continued to climb, Congress attempted to reassert its control over public assistance and to place a cap on welfare benefits. Grants to families in which the father had died and grants to families with unemployed fathers continued as open-ended entitlements. Congress "froze" the level of federal grants for cases attributable to desertion or illegitimacy. Asked Wilbur Mills rhetorically, "Is it in the public interest for welfare to become a way of life?"

In 1935, having children without fathers, their mothers, old people, and blind people dependent on welfare as a way of life had served the public interest; in 1967, welfare was considered a temporary way station, a place for a disadvantaged or discouraged person to gather skills or courage. The notion of mothers' pensions, keeping widows at home with their children, no longer described welfare programs or defined the terms of welfare practice. Between 1935 and 1967, welfare, once a do-good program conducted in a nonpartisan manner, became the object of a highly contentious debate over what the next generation of policy analysts would call welfare reform.

---

6   Welfare Restated, 1967–1988

If there was a difference between welfare reform before and after 1967, it concerned an important change in the profession of the reformers. Before 1967, social workers dominated the debate; economists became increasingly prominent after 1967.

Social workers equated social policy and individual therapy. Through an intensive application of sheer manpower and effective expertise, the nation could win the war on poverty, allowing the social welfare system to function in the grand style of the postwar consensus in which social insurance solved most people's problems and social workers attended to the problems of the few who remained outside of the labor force. Although the Newburgh situation and growing disclosures of welfare chiselers exposed dissatisfaction with the grand design in the early 1960s, the booming economy and the promises that policy analysts made to politicians tended to dispel doubts. The nation could face its welfare problems with full confidence that the welfare rate would eventually yield to the time and attention that experts lavished upon it. Indeed, the abolition of poverty itself lay well within the nation's capabilities.

In a few years, these hopes dissipated, and economists replaced the social workers in the front lines of welfare reform and the war on poverty. Confidence, in this area of policy as in Social Security, yielded to crisis; consensus gave way to conflict over the best approach to follow. The rehabilitation strategy appeared to fall apart. Urban riots, among other domestic developments, mocked the planners' desires to build stronger communities in the inner cities. On

April 4, 1968, for example, the death of Martin Luther King, himself a spokesman for nonviolence, interracial accommodation, and integration, spawned a nationwide series of riots in which thirty-seven people died.

A perceived link between domestic and foreign events intensified the sense of failure. General William C. Westmoreland, returning from a tour of duty in Vietnam, reflected that downtown Washington in the aftermath of Dr. King's assassination "looked considerably more distressing than Saigon during the Tet offensive." The nation felt burned by both events. The Tet offensive, a January 1968 North Vietnamese campaign that brought the enemy to the gates of the American embassy in Saigon, surprised the military leadership and shocked the American public. It made many Americans realize that the nation might not "win" the Vietnam War. As historian Kim McQuaid has written, "Tet made it appear that the emperors had no clothes, or far fewer than they had claimed." Urban riots, in a similar sense, stripped social policy theorists of their cloak of legitimacy and increased the odds against winning the war on poverty.

Policymakers responded similarly to both events, initiating a process of disengagement. The height of American casualties in the Vietnam war came in 1968. After that date, policymakers attempted to substitute South Vietnamese soldiers for American soldiers, South Vietnamese casualties for American deaths. The United States maintained its commitment but at a distance, turning from face-to-face combat to the automated battlefield, in which, as McQuaid notes, war became "increasingly dynamic, technological, and fought by remote control." Between the summer of 1967 and the spring of 1968, racial confrontation in America's cities reached its height. After those months, policymakers began to pull the social workers out of the ghettos and to substitute money for services as the primary tool of the war on poverty. In place of intensive individual therapy, policymakers now turned to a more automated, less discretionary form of mass social action.

The change made a difference in the way welfare was perceived. Social workers had tried to adjust the psychology of the individual; economists, assuming away psychological problems, replaced individual pathology with economic rationality. They assumed a world in which people responded rationally to economic incentives. Where social workers wanted to adjust individual psyches, economists hoped to change the nature of the choices offered by public policy.

The Coming and Going of the Family Assistance Plan

The first inkling of a policy change came in the last days of the Johnson administration. The president, despairing of urban violence and other forms of domestic discord, turned, as he often did, to the advice of outside experts. At the beginning of 1968, still thinking of himself as a possible candidate in that fall's election, he appointed a presidential commission to investigate income maintenance programs. The commission's report, which made its public debut in 1969 after Johnson had dropped out of the race and Richard Nixon had already become president, suggested a new formulation of the liberal position on welfare, a retreat from rehabilitation to work incentives.

The report implied that very few of the poor were shiftless people trapped within a culture of poverty. Far from needing rehabilitation to acquire a will to work, they wanted to get jobs, but too often they discovered that they could make more money by going on welfare. The report called on the government to replace the system that required withdrawal from the labor force as a condition of government aid with one that encouraged welfare recipients to work. Boldly suggesting scrapping the present welfare system, the report recommended substituting a guaranteed income of $2400 and building onto that guarantee substantial incentives that would make it profitable for people to work.

Even in 1969, work incentives played a part in the AFDC program. Far from sympathetic to abolishing the AFDC program and reluctant to abandon the rehabilitation approach, Johnson administration officials still recognized the value of removing work disincentives from the program. In 1967, Wilbur Cohen, at the time the undersecretary of Health, Education, and Welfare, negotiated with Congress an "earnings disregard." Although expressed in technical terms, the concept relied on the simple notion of allowing welfare recipients to keep some of the money they earned from working. Before 1967, working welfare recipients had faced severe penalties. For each dollar they earned, local authorities reduced their welfare checks by a dollar. A woman who received $90 from welfare and earned $90 from working gained nothing: if she worked, she received $90 from her job but lost that much in welfare, if she stayed home, she received $90 from the local welfare agency. After 1967, a welfare mother got to keep the first $30 she made each month, and one-third of the remainder of her earnings. A woman who received $90 from welfare and earned $90 from working gained $50: the initial $30 of her earnings that she got to keep plus one-third of the remainder of her earnings—one third of $60 equals $20. If she worked, she received $50 from welfare and

$90 from working for a total of $140. If she stayed home, she received $90 from welfare.

Even this simple illustration demonstrates that, as the Johnson administration strove to make the welfare program more modern and efficient, it also increased the program's complexity. Working through even the simplest examples caused most people's eyes to glaze over.

The President's Commission on Income Maintenance proposed an even more complex program, with both a guaranteed income, for someone earning nothing, and a work disregard (or, in the technical jargon, a marginal tax rate below 1), for low-income workers. The commission's staff members manipulated these sorts of concepts and proposals with a fluid ease since, as economists, they fluently spoke the language of applied social policy. In 1961, when Ribicoff and Kennedy planned their version of welfare reform, they relied on the advice of social workers, who staffed the 1961 Ad Hoc Committee on Public Welfare; now the economists entered the discussion, and soon took center stage. In various think tanks and government bureaus, they continued to influence the welfare reform debate.

Although the report of the President's Commission on Income Maintenance would be opposed by the Nixon administration as the work of the Johnson administration and was ignored by important figures within the Johnson administration, who disapproved of abandoning the rehabilitation approach and eliminating AFDC, it nonetheless foreshadowed an important policy shift. Richard M. Nixon, not burdened by loyalty to the policies of Presidents Roosevelt and Kennedy, absorbed the commission's report and made a sweeping welfare proposal of his own, known as the Family Assistance Plan (FAP).

Nixon drew on three arguments in the economists' arsenal to criticize the existing welfare system and to design his own plan. First, welfare discouraged work. By working, a woman might well reduce her total income; industrious and intelligent women, imbued with a capitalistic desire to maximize their incomes, stayed out of the labor force.

Second, cash grants put more money into a woman's pocket than therapy or other services did. "The curse of the poor," argued Nobel laureate economist Paul Samuelson, "is literally their poverty. Give them more money and not only they but their progeny can break through the vicious cycle."

Third, welfare destroyed the nuclear family. Because many states limited AFDC payments to families without fathers and all states prohibited payments to families with a working father, the AFDC program encouraged husbands to desert their wives and pregnant mothers to remain unmarried. If a man who earned $2.00 an hour decided to leave his wife and two children, the annual income of the woman and children he left behind would increase by an average of $2,158. Assuming that the man's income remained constant, the family would do much better split up than together, much better on welfare than off the rolls. A Minnesota mother of three would receive welfare benefits until her income reached $8,000 a year, unless of course the father remained in the house, in which case the family would fail to qualify for any welfare benefits. Unless the man earned substantially more than $8,000, a rational, capitalistic, profit-maximizing couple would stay apart.

Together, these arguments defined the welfare problem and pointed toward its solution. One could increase work incentives and strengthen family structures by letting welfare recipients keep more of their earnings and by not restricting welfare payments to single-parent families. One could accomplish these goals more efficiently through cash payments than through services.

Nixon, impressed by these arguments but wary of expanding the nation's social welfare programs, made welfare an immediate priority of his new administration. As Nixon later recalled, he wanted to get rid of the "costly failures of the Great Society," and he regarded the welfare system as the "worst offender." He quickly set members of his administration to devising the Nixon welfare reform plan, only to discover considerable disarray within his administration. On one side stood Daniel Patrick Moynihan and the innovators, ready with a radical proposal. On the other side stood the traditionalists who opposed a plan that paid welfare to the working poor.

Daniel Patrick Moynihan, as much as anyone, defined the course of the welfare reform debate over the course of the next twenty years. When Moynihan was 10, his father, a newspaper reporter, deserted the family. Moving from place to place, Moynihan managed to attend City College for a year before he entered the navy. Leaving naval service in 1947, he studied at Tufts University on the GI bill and helped his mother run a saloon in the Hell's Kitchen neighborhood of Manhattan. A Democrat, like nearly everyone else in the neighborhood, he began his political career in state government, working for New York's Governor Averell Harriman in the 1950s, before concentrating on graduate school.

Moynihan's New York political contacts helped him land a job in the Kennedy administration, first as an assistant to Secretary of Labor Arthur Goldberg and then as an assistant secretary of labor in charge of planning and development. His position gave him considerable opportunity to ruminate on the problems of the day and led him to produce a report in 1965 that acquired wide notoriety and exerted an important influence over the welfare reform debate. It became known as the Moynihan report.

In *The Negro Family: The Case for National Action*, Moynihan argued that the unstable black family contributed to "welfare and crime and welfare dependence." He amassed considerable evidence to demonstrate this instability: nearly a quarter of urban black marriages were dissolved; nearly a quarter of black births were illegitimate; nearly a quarter of black families were headed by a female. The instability of the family undermined the position of the males within it. Lacking a stable place within the economic system and constructive role models, black men failed to become strong husbands and fathers. In this way they contributed to a never-ending cycle of family breakup that was a central feature of what Moynihan called the "tangle of pathology" of the urban ghetto. "In essence," he wrote, "the Negro family has been forced into a matriarchal society which, because it is so out of line with the rest of American society, seriously retards the progress of the group as a whole and imposes a crushing burden on the Negro male and, in consequence, on a great many Negro women as well."

If this pathology were ever to be cured, Moynihan suggested, the government would have to direct its attention to the black family. In particular, it needed to promote a family structure that gave the male more of a place within the family, so that black males would learn how to provide for their families. Once this fundamental change in family structure was accomplished, then the other elements in the civil rights strategy—the promotion of legal rights and the provision of job training—would begin to be effective. As long as the "Negro family in the urban ghettos is crumbling," Moynihan believed, "the programs that have been enacted in the first phase of the Negro revolution . . . only make opportunities available. They cannot insure the outcome."

The Moynihan report represented a call to action that almost no one heeded, because it rubbed nearly everyone the wrong way. Black leaders, achieving influence in Washington for the first time in a century, saw little advantage to calling attention to tangles of social pathology. After the 1965 Watts riots, as confrontation replaced interracial cooperation, black leaders proved even more reluctant to focus attention on shortcomings within the black community. Liberals, at the height of their optimism over the government's ability to improve social conditions, thought that making opportunities available was the right course to follow, regardless of Moynihan's warnings about the black family.

Liberal scholars skewered Moynihan, objecting to his right to sit in judgment of the black family and to his implicit point that families headed by males provided society with more economic benefits than female-headed families. It was an era in which whites, despite the liberal optimism about improving social conditions, lacked confidence in their dealings with blacks. Some scholars wrote that Moynihan, failing to appreciate the strength and diversity of the black family, suffered from a form of ethnic hubris that labeled deviations from white, middle-class standards as pathologies. Anthropologist Carol Stack accused Moynihan of remaining trapped within conventional definitions of the family and thus misunderstanding what Michael Katz describes as the "domestic experience of poor black Americans." Historians, notably Herbert Gutman, also faulted the report, arguing that, depending on outdated sources, Moynihan had gotten his facts wrong, particularly on the history of the black family.

Further, Moynihan, although a brilliant synthesizer, had produced his report quickly and had sometimes let his eye for the persuasive anecdote grow larger than his stomach for elaborate social science methodology. Academics believed that the report, like its author, was too flamboyant, too careless with the exceptions to general rules that, for the academics, often became matters that consumed entire careers.

Moynihan, who managed to secure a position at Harvard after his government service in the Kennedy and Johnson administrations, felt stung by the liberal criticism of his report. Liberals, who prided themselves on their realism, refused to relinquish a romantic view of blacks as somehow morally superior to whites. This romanticism blinded them to the problems of the ghetto and left them unprepared for the violence of the middle 1960s. When Leonard Garment, a former Nixon law partner, worked to secure a position for Moynihan in the Nixon administration, Moynihan encouraged his efforts, hoping to demonstrate that the conservatives could succeed at fundamental social reform where the liberals had produced only confrontation and resentment. He therefore entered the Nixon White House as a domestic advisor to the President.

As Moynihan joined the White House staff, he allied himself with a group of liberals, who began to rethink the fundamental assumptions of the Kennedy and Johnson years and who became dubbed neoconservatives. A product of the working class, Moynihan, in common with a long line of American self-made politicians that began with Alexander Hamilton, feared the collapse of social order. The urban riots of the 1960s appeared to Moynihan to indicate a breakdown in civility and to pose a dangerous threat to social stability.

The solution, he came to believe, involved not the empowerment of people in the ghetto so much as practical benefits to help people leave the ghetto. Income and jobs, reinforced by strong families, topped the list.

Moynihan, a man of considerable wit and charm, described by one of his competitors on the White House staff as a "playful porpoise," sent the president a series of memos on ways to end what Nixon called the "welfare mess." An Anglophile who had attended the London School of Economics on a Fulbright scholarship, Moynihan cast Nixon in the role of Benjamin Disraeli, the conservative prime minister who had seen the cohesive value of social reform amid the squalor of Victorian England. Nixon, in Moynihan's hopeful vision, held the power to ameliorate social conditions in the manner of Disraeli and strengthen the conservative institutions of home and family.

The traditionalists, who opposed Moynihan and deeply distrusted his motives, portrayed him as a Democratic interloper in a conservative administration. They argued against expanding the welfare state and for a return to the traditional system as it had functioned in 1935. Arthur Burns, an economist from Columbia University, who was Nixon's chief economic advisor in the 1960 campaign and a personal friend, warned against "moving away from the concept of welfare based on disability-related deprivation and need to the concept of welfare as a matter of right." Burns favored raising benefits for the deserving poor, those excused from the labor force, and opposed extending welfare to the working poor.

Like Moynihan and the innovators, the traditionalists used economics to argue their case. What the outcome would be of giving welfare to people already working and not presently on welfare remained unclear. Someone already working might discover that he could increase his income by ceasing to work and opting for leisure. Suppose, for example, that the plan guaranteed a minimum income of $3,000 and that someone working full time made $2,500. A person who stopped working altogether would receive a bonus of $500. Rules requiring the person to work often proved impossible to enforce.

Getting the man to continue his job with incentives such as those contemplated by the innovators presented difficult, perhaps insurmountable technical problems. The major incentive proposed by the innovators consisted of allowing a person to keep a share of his earnings without penalty. In one variation of the plan, for example, the government would permit the man to keep half of his earnings and still receive the minimum benefit. The man earning $2,500 "kept" $1,250. Since, according to the terms of the previous example, he also received a guarantee of $3,000, his after-tax income and his guarantee would total $4,250. His working therefore increased his income by $1250. The traditionalists proceeded to ask, Would such a person maintain his level of work effort for this extra money, or would he elect, in the economists' terms, to consume more leisure? The traditionalists feared that such a person would cut back on the number of hours he worked. The work incentives would have failed, the government's expenditures would increase, and the welfare problem would remain as pressing as ever.

After listening to the arguments, Nixon endorsed the Family Assistance Plan because he saw great advantages to a cash, as opposed to a service, strategy. "I thought," he later wrote, "that people should have the responsibility for spending carefully and taking care of themselves. I abhorred snoopy, patronizing surveillance by social workers which made children and adults feel stigmatized and separate. The basic premise of the Family Assistance Plan was simple: what the poor need to help them rise out of poverty is money." Nixon realized that many of these snoopy social workers perpetuated pork-barrel programs in Democratic districts. If anything, they strengthened the Democrat's hold on inner cities. Moynihan encouraged Nixon in his distrust of social workers. Returning from a crucial meeting on the welfare reform plan, Moynihan characterized it as "a good meeting, a very good meeting with Nixon. The president asked me, 'Will FSS (an early acronym for the welfare reform plan) get rid of social workers?' and I promised him it would wipe them out." In this manner, philosophy and politics reinforced one another, and the innovators carried the day.

For Nixon, Moynihan's invitation proved irresistible, despite the objections of the traditionalists. Proposing a new system that emphasized work rather than welfare, families rather than single mothers, allowed Nixon to dismantle the flawed program of Roosevelt, Kennedy, and Johnson and replace it with his own, superior creation.

Nixon unveiled his Family Assistance Plan on August 8, 1969. His announcement came a few days after an American walked on the moon and toward the end of the season that was later referred to as the "Woodstock summer," in honor of a mass gathering of young people in an upstate New York meadow to attend a rock and roll concert and enjoy one another's company. Two images stuck in the public's mind: the nation's technological capability, which orchestrated the impressive moon launch, and the hedonism of the young who arrogantly proclaimed themselves a separate nation, one dedicated to drugs, sex, and rock and roll. During this summer, a stolid Richard Nixon, broadcasting from an Oval Office deliberately kept at frigid temperatures, reminded Americans of the virtues of work and family and promised a technological breakthrough on the domestic front to match the moon walk.

The plan Nixon proposed contained a guaranteed annual income of $1600 for a family of four, a $720 work disregard, and a marginal tax rate of 50 percent. These technical terms meant nothing to Nixon's television audience, and the administration developed accompanying proposals for food stamps that made the total package even more complicated. Few people appreciated the radical nature of the proposal. Unlike Presidents Roosevelt, Truman, Eisenhower, Kennedy and Johnson, President Richard M. Nixon wanted to abolish Aid to Families with Dependent Children and to substitute for it a program that reached working families with children.

An appreciation of Nixon's proposal required policymakers in Congress to receive intensive instruction in the design of social policy, and few appeared eager to master the details. Representative Barber Conable, the influential New York Republican and participant in the 1983 Social Security compromise, once remarked that successful programs were ones that could be reduced to slogans that fit on bumper stickers. The Family Assistance Plan failed this pragmatic test. The easiest example through which to understand the program concerned a family with two children and two unemployed parents. The family received from the federal government the basic guarantee of $1,600 or about $133 a month. That looked like a small amount of money until one considered that such a family might previously have received nothing from the government, if, for example, the father had exhausted his unemployment benefits and the state in which the family lived did not participate in the welfare program for unemployed fathers.

In addition, the Nixon administration proposed that such a family should also receive food stamps, special vouchers good only for food items. The rules for computing food stamp benefits lay beyond most people's comprehension. They involved the notion that a family should need to spend only 30 percent of its income on a minimum adequate diet. At the time, such a diet cost, according to the Department of Agriculture, $1200 a year for a family of four. Hence, the rules required families that received $1600 from the government under FAP to spend 30 percent of their income on food. That amounted to $480. In exchange for this $480, the family received food stamps worth $1200 that they could take to the grocery store and spend on food. That represented a "bonus" of $720 ($1200 − $480) that the family received from food stamps. Hence, a family of four, with two unemployed parents, received the equivalent of $2320 under the Nixon proposal. Expressed in 1990 dollars, that amounted to about

$7,000 a year, not a great amount, to be sure, but nonetheless more than such a family might have received before.

Many families, of course, contained working fathers, and such families were the real targets of Nixon's proposal. Here the other features of the plan came into play. Assume, for example, a family of four in which the father earned $3,000. Under the Nixon rules, the father "kept" the first $720 under the work disregard rule. That left $2,280 subject to the 50 percent tax, which amounted to $1,140. This family therefore received the guarantee of $1600, the work disregard of $720, and the after-tax earnings of $1,140 for a total of $3,460. But the father was already earning $3,000, so the government sent the father a check for $460, plus an additional food stamp "bonus" of $162.

The complicated nature of the plan and the difficulties of coordinating it with existing programs added to its political liabilities and contributed to its ultimate defeat. Although FAP passed the House, it ran into substantial problems, which produced its defeat, in the Senate. Simply put, the plan failed to satisfy people on the right or people on the left. On the right, it encountered the sorts of arguments that Burns had advanced within the administration. Conservatives portrayed FAP as expensive, since it would cost at least $4 billion a year, and as a dangerous expansion of welfare for the working poor.

Liberals objected to the Family Assistance Plan for more complicated reasons. Because of the technical complexity, the plan lacked a ready means of comparison with existing programs. The easiest number on which to focus was the guarantee to a family of four with two unemployed parents of $1600 a year. That number looked low, and liberals, who distrusted Nixon and did not wish to lose their role as prime policy innovators, could easily outbid Nixon on it. As liberals raised the guarantee, however, the potential cost began to balloon, because of the program's true nature as aid to the working poor, not just the unemployed. Once the government started to pay benefits to the broad middle class, even small benefits, costs would rise astronomically because of the sheer number of people who would be receiving benefits.

Here another iron law of social policy to match the iron law of rising pension costs exercised its tyranny. It held that raising the guarantee and maintaining the same "tax" on benefits automatically raised the "break-even" point, the point at which the government stopped paying benefits. Indeed, a multiplier effect occurred. A guarantee of $3,000 and a tax of 50 percent implied a break-even point of $6,000. Raise the guarantee by a thousand dollars and one increased the break-even point by $2,000. Hence, a bidding war on the government's guarantee carried deceptively high costs.

The notion of the break-even point, like so much else about the proposal, was a difficult one for the policymakers to grasp. A guarantee of $1,600 and a tax rate of 50 percent implied a break-even point of $3,200 (assuming, for the sake of simplicity, no work disregard). Someone who earned $3,200 would not receive anything from the government. Why? The person who earned $3,200 was guaranteed $1,600 and half of his earnings (also $1600), for a total of $3,200. But that person already made $3,200; hence the government owed him nothing.

The break-even point led to yet another problem that exposed political liabilities of the plan and produced both liberal and conservative opposition. Economists, who found the entire FAP exercise to be a stimulating mental puzzle, referred to "notch" effects that created work disincentives. Comprehending the situation required the ability to think like an economist. Consider, as in the example, a break-even point of $3200. Now, throw in a rule that says that only people on welfare can get health insurance for free. That means that a person making $3,000 receives health insurance at no cost to himself, and a person making $3,200 has to pay for his own health insurance. (Remember that the person making $3,200 was ineligible for welfare.) Now, tote up the benefits. The person making $3,000 would have a total income of $3100, including $100 from the government, and free health insurance. He got the extra $100 from the government because he was guaranteed $1,600, plus half of his earnings, $1,500, for a total of $3,100. Since he made only $3,000, the government owed him the extra hundred. He got health insurance because he was still on welfare. The person making $3200 received $3200 but no free health insurance. If the cash value of the health insurance was more than $100, the person without welfare ended up worse off than the person on welfare. That meant that the plan contained a hidden work disincentive.

Similar defects appeared during the Senate Finance Committee hearings on FAP in April 1970. Senator John Williams, a conservative Republican from Delaware who did not plan to seek reelection, presided over a demonstration of notch effects, using charts prepared for him by the Department of Health, Education, and Welfare. The charts showed that, under the president's plan, a welfare mother in Chicago who made $720 a year ended up with $6,128 a year, in the form of cash, public housing, food stamps, and medical care. A mother in similar circumstances who earned $5,560 received a total of only

$6,109. The welfare mother who showed initiative and attempted to work her way off welfare ended up $19 dollars poorer for her efforts. In other words, the president's plan failed to eliminate the work disincentives that adhered to the welfare system. Further, getting rid of all of these disincentives meant changing most of the programs that interacted with welfare, wiping the slate clean, and encountering insuperable political difficulties, as defenders of the various programs protected their turf.

The Nixon administration tried to cope with the now obvious enormous problems of social design inherent in the Family Assistance Plan, only to be severely criticized once again from the left. Liberal sentiments culminated in self-proclaimed "people's hearings," held in November 1970, in which Senator Eugene McCarthy (D-Minn.) took testimony from what journalist Mary McGrory described as "scores of militant welfare mothers" who "bellowed their opposition to being driven out of the house to do underpaid work." George Wiley of the National Welfare Rights Organization attended the hearings, dressed in a colorful African dashiki. Objecting to the work provisions that the Nixon administration had attached to the bill, he insisted on an absolute guarantee with no work requirements. Wiley argued for the dignity of welfare mothers by demeaning Richard Nixon in the confrontational rhetoric of the era: "You don't promote family life by forcing women out of their homes to empty bedpans. When Richard Nixon is ready to give up his $200,000 salary to scrub floors and empty bedpans in the interest of his family, then we will take him seriously." This scene did not sit well with the conservative members of the Senate Finance Committee, who shortly thereafter voted against FAP, nor with Richard Nixon, who failed to support subsequent attempts by Abraham Ribicoff, now a Connecticut senator, to revive the idea.

President Nixon, an extraordinarily difficult man to analyze, may have preferred the image of noble failure to that of mere participant in a brokered victory for which the Democrats would take much of the credit. In domestic policy, with Congress under tight Democratic control, Nixon lacked the means to impose his will, as Franklin Roosevelt and Lyndon Johnson had done. Thus, Nixon faced a much harder time overcoming demagoguery on the FAP proposal than FDR had on the Social Security bill. The attacks were similar. Just as FDR had offered a "pauper's dole" to the elderly, so President Nixon wanted to shortchange welfare mothers, throw them out of the house, and make them work.

In the end, Congress opted for reform along the lines originally suggested by Arthur Burns. In October 1972, it raised benefits for the "deserving" poor and created the Supplemental Security Income (SSI)

The Frustrations of Welfare Reform

program. For the first time, the federal government supported an absolute monthly guarantee of $210 for an elderly couple on welfare. And not only did SSI cover the elderly, it also covered the blind and the permanently and totally disabled. Further, the federal government, rather than the states, would administer SSI. It therefore represented a major change in welfare policy that, in the midst of the FAP debate, went almost unnoticed. Similar liberalizations of the food stamp program, along the lines proposed by President Nixon, also attracted little attention, even as they raised welfare benefits, reduced differentials in benefits from place to place, and strengthened federal administrative control over the system.

It looked like progress, even if the Family Assistance Program had failed, yet it reflected a troublesome social judgment. Passage of SSI meant that the deserving poor would not have to go to state and local government offices but rather, like Social Security beneficiaries, could receive their checks in the mail. Policymakers created the program with the elderly in mind, yet the disabled soon became the program's primary beneficiaries. In December 1984, for example, 2.4 million disabled people and 1.5 million aged people received SSI. Although disabled persons could receive government assistance, linking benefits to an inability to work mitigated against their efforts at rehabilitation and finding a job. In a sense, it consigned them to a benevolent trap that, as the capabilities of people with handicaps increased, grew deeper and deeper.

It seemed that the only thing that the government could handle well was paying people to retire. Plans for the rehabilitation of AFDC beneficiaries lurched along in the usual uncertain manner and the rolls continued to expand. In 1971, Congress, faced with the fourth straight year of double-digit increases in the percentage growth of the AFDC caseload, enacted the "Talmadge Amendments," named for Senator Herman Talmadge (D-Ga.). These required AFDC recipients who were not caring for children under six to register for the Work Incentive Program (WIN), which had been created in 1967. That nicely expressed the state of welfare policy in the 1970s: the deserving poor received a guaranteed income; AFDC recipients, now firmly entrenched as the undeserving poor, endured what came to be known as workfare.

Workfare

A year after President Nixon endorsed the Family Assistance Plan, Governor Ronald Reagan of California sent a letter to his cabinet in which he announced the formation of a task force to examine public assistance. This task force hoped to produce a plan that would put a stop to the growth of the state's welfare rolls, then increasing at the rate of 40,000 AFDC recipients a month. Reagan wanted to reduce the number on the rolls by "purifying" the welfare system and limiting welfare to those "strictly entitled." In this regard, Reagan followed a line similar to that of Arthur Burns and the traditionalists advising President Nixon. Like Burns, Reagan wanted to maintain welfare for the "truly needy" but require others to work in order to survive.

Calling the welfare system "a moral and administrative disaster," Reagan presented his welfare reform plan to the California legislature on March 3, 1971. The plan relied on trimming ineligible people from the welfare rolls, on forcing fathers and other relatives to assume responsibility for dependent children, and on making the able-bodied poor work for their grants. Reagan explained that the system was designed to give back to the truly needy the dignity of which they had been robbed by people who had defrauded the public and slipped onto the welfare rolls. The presence of these chiselers on the welfare rolls swelled the state's tax bills, and the taxpayers, as Reagan put it, refused to "foot the bill" for "providing benefits to millions not in need."

Reagan explicitly objected to the concept of a guaranteed income. In the first place, he did not think that the solution to the welfare problem should come from the federal government, because that would prevent society from remaining "responsive and flexible." Federal programs inevitably involved, according to Reagan, "massive bureaucratic structures" that hardened into "self-perpetuating" entities. In the second place, the guaranteed income, far from preserving work incentives, actually destroyed them. "What incentive is there for quality or quantity in work or employment if a guaranteed income is created?" asked Governor Reagan.

The California plan achieved modest reductions in the numbers of people served by the Aid to Families with Dependent Children program. In May 1971, the California AFDC rolls contained 1,285,742 people (excluding those in the unemployed parent segment of the program); in June 1972, 1,270,907 people remained on the rolls. The California experience resembled that of New York, in which the number of welfare recipients peaked in 1972, even though Nelson Rockefeller, New York's governor, took no special steps to reduce the growth of the rolls. The largest rate of increase in crucially important New York City came in 1968, well before both Nixon's and Reagan's proposals. Further, the caseworkers administering Reagan's plan reacted ambivalently to it, some no doubt feeling like their colleagues in New York. There, according to Blanche Bernstein, a former New

The Frustrations of Welfare Reform

York City welfare administrator, "it became something of a badge of honor for caseworkers to manipulate the regulations to build the largest possible grant for a client." Despite these facts, California officials boomed the plan, which they claimed had stemmed the growth of welfare. "California's welfare system can become a model for the nation," said Robert Carleson, Reagan's state social welfare director.

An important part of the model involved workfare. In a sense, traditionalists like Reagan considered a work requirement to be the logical counterpart to the innovators' offer of a minimum income. People, they assumed, wanted to work, and those capable of working welcomed the prospect of paying off their welfare grants through public service. In Reagan's Community Work Experience Program, welfare recipients worked for as many hours as it took to pay off their welfare grants at the minimum wage.

Reagan thought of workfare as a form of compulsion, as an obligation on the part of the poor to the community, and as a form of deterrent. If someone wanted to go on welfare, the work requirement might help dissuade him from applying. Reagan tended to discount other benefits that might accrue from the program, such as skills that the worker might acquire.

Although Ronald Reagan held few illusions about the uplifting nature of workfare, his program still foundered on the realities of the job market. Workfare participants received the minimum wage. Relatively low welfare grants and comparatively high minimum wages meant that it did not take long for a welfare recipient to pay off her welfare grant. No one needed to work forty hour weeks for a whole month in order to pay off the grant.

Nationwide, workfare ran into similar problems, which called the utility of the approach into question. Beginning in 1971, Congress required able-bodied welfare recipients to register for the Work Incentive Program, but few welfare recipients fell into the eligible categories. After children, the elderly, the blind, disabled persons, and mothers of children under the age of six were eliminated from the list, few welfare recipients remained. The fact that the Department of Labor and the Department of Health, Education, and Welfare jointly administered the Work Incentive Program at the federal level added to the complications, as did the fact that each state maintained a separate unit within its welfare department to run the program. It amounted to a cumbersome, frequently contentious bureaucratic arrangement.

The WIN program ended up serving a very small percentage of welfare mothers and fathers. In December 1974, for example, 3.3

million heads of households received AFDC, of whom 1.3 million registered for WIN. For various administrative reasons, authorities selected fewer than a quarter of a million people to participate in the program. The total number of participants, including those selected in previous years, amounted to a little more than half a million. The federal government appropriated $340 million for the program in fiscal 1974, or about $680 for each participant. Even before they joined the program, more than half of those who participated in the program in 1974 required subsidized child care. Of the approximately 500,000 participants in the WIN program in 1974, about a third took jobs in what program administrators called "unsubsidized employment," predominantly in service, semiskilled, and unskilled occupations. Of the group that started jobs, about a third quit within 90 days. Fifty-two thousand people left the welfare rolls. The federal government therefore spent more than $6,800 for each person who left the rolls, with little assurance that they would not be back.

Experimenting with Guaranteed Income

As policymakers puzzled over what to do about workfare, social scientists decided to put the guaranteed annual income to the test. They conducted vigorous experiments that would answer many of the remaining questions. In particular, they wanted to determine how people would respond to this income. What if, in the style of the television program in which the host gave a person a million dollars, the government simply offered a guaranteed annual income to a family? Would family members reduce the number of hours they worked? If a person knew that she could get welfare, regardless of her marital condition, what would happen to family stability? Would there be more marriages or more divorces? Social scientists hoped to take such questions beyond ideology and politics and come up with impartial, scientifically determined answers, using actual communities operating under real conditions as the laboratories. The income maintenance experiments, as they came to be called, marked the zenith of the economist's influence over the welfare reform debate.

Although the scope of the experiments was impressive, the results only confused the welfare reform debate further. The federal government undertook four large-scale experiments in the late 1960s and the 1970s. These included one in Trenton, New Jersey, that involved 1,357 households and enabled analysts to focus on declining urban areas. Another experiment concerned rural areas, and a third experiment concentrated on black households in Gary, Indiana. The final experiment, which took place in Seattle and Denver between

1971 and 1982, allowed social scientists to look at a relatively large sample of 4,800 families for an extended period of time.

The first news from the experiments cheered the proponents of a guaranteed annual income. Partial results from the New Jersey experiment in February 1970 suggested that work effort did not decline among people receiving income support payments. These results soon made their way into congressional deliberation over FAP: evidence that a guaranteed income would not destroy work incentives.

More of the data, however, brought different news. As economists studied the results, they discovered what many of them had suspected: a guaranteed income reduced work effort. As the government gave money to the working poor, the family members adjusted by working fewer hours. Hence, much of the money spent for a guaranteed annual income actually replaced money that the families had previously raised by working. Economist Alicia Munnell estimated that as much as half of the government's money would be spent with this result.

The data also brought surprising and distressing news from the experiment conducted in Seattle and Denver. A guaranteed income offered to two-parent and one-parent families increased the rate at which marriages dissolved by 40 to 60 percent. Henry Aaron, a Brookings Institution economist, said that the "apparent discrepancy between common sense and experimental results was as dramatic as any that have been realized through social science research." If these results were true, it meant that the notion that welfare broke up families by forcing wives and husbands to separate or by discouraging pregnant women from getting married amounted to mere propaganda, unsupported by science. Give people a choice between accepting welfare in one-parent or in two-parent families, and they responded by getting divorced and forming one-parent families.

But were the results true? The computer could dissect the data in all sorts of ways. Whites and Hispanics apparently reacted differently than did black families. Among whites the "effect" of family break-up stopped in the second year and reversed in the third. The effect among Hispanics never acquired "statistical significance." Only among blacks did the effect continue for three years. To say the least, the results generated confusion, as policymakers hastened to know the truth, only to be told by the social scientists that the truth could not be reduced to a simple yes or no answer.

As Munnell noted, the "very rigor" of the experiments limited their "policy relevance." The results needed to be qualified in all sorts of ways, adjusted to reflect the limited number of plans tested, differences in results among the experiments, softness in the data caused by people reporting their income level or hours of work incorrectly, and the number of people who disappeared from the sample. Such qualifications bred intramural arguments among the economists who knew econometric techniques and could speak the language of social science. Such people, who lived apart from ordinary citizens in what political scientist Hugh Heclo termed "splendid isolation," soon found themselves talking mainly to each other. When the policymakers asked the economists questions, the economists told the policymakers both too much and too little.

Even though the babble of social science raised as many questions as it answered and the results of workfare programs proved disappointing, politicians continued to tackle welfare reform throughout the 1970s. In reality, three approaches, the community action/service approach, workfare, and a guaranteed annual income, surfaced in the sixties and seventies, but none appeared to hold the answer. Nothing, it seemed, could force welfare recipients to work.

As time passed, the problem became progressively worse. Although each president tried to reform the welfare system in a grand manner, each succeeded only in chipping away a little of the old system and replacing it with something new. The more pieces there were in place, the more difficult the task of comprehensive reform became.

The President's Commission for a National Agenda for the Eighties, convened by Jimmy Carter in 1979, captured the growing sense of futility that accompanied discussions of welfare. First, the commission learned of the labyrinthine welfare bureaucracy. In some cases, it took fourteen hundred pieces of information just to determine a person's income level. A recently widowed mother of several children, one of whom was disabled, would have to go to four different offices, fill out five different forms, and answer three hundred separate questions in order to receive aid. The Carter administration resented the inefficiency of such a system, yet could do little about it, since control over welfare programs lay divided among sixty congressional committees and subcommittees.

Part of the problem stemmed from the fact that public officials held welfare recipients to higher standards than those followed by the rest of the community, creating what Blanche Bernstein described as an "Alice in Wonderland-ish quality." Most working mothers made do with existing child care provisions; but "once the mother is on welfare," wrote Bernstein, "she cannot work unless a variety of officials agree that the child care arrangements are satisfactory." In a similar manner, officials expected welfare recipients not to have to put up with contradictory pieces of advice, long waits in government offices,

The Frustrations of Welfare Reform

and confusing rules for calculating assets, yet other citizens often received conflicting pieces of advice, waited hours in doctor's offices, and puzzled over their bank statements. Indeed, the very fact that the welfare system contained so many facets often worked to the advantage of welfare recipients, rather than to their disadvantage. As Bernstein noted, New York officials routinely understated the size of the average welfare grant in New York City in the 1970s by reporting only the basic grant and omitting rent subsidies, food stamps, free school lunches, a fuel allowance, and subsidized medical care. If one added these things, the average total grant amounted to 88 percent of the Bureau of Labor Statistics lower level budget, well above the income that a minimum wage job provided for a family of four in 1981.

Members of President Carter's commission learned first-hand of the frustrations of the welfare system when they traveled to Chicago in 1980 to hear the testimony of welfare recipients who regarded the aid they were receiving as dangerously inadequate to meet their needs. At the time, an Illinois family on welfare might have received $500 a month. By this time, the welfare recipients deeply resented the continuing presence of blue-ribbon panels that professed great concern for their plight, took considerable testimony, and never returned. The Chicago hearing became confrontational, as one member of the audience demanded to know how many of the commissioners had ever been on welfare.

There was growing frustration on the part of both policymakers, who, like New York's Blanche Bernstein, were beginning to rethink their commitment to welfare as a form of social melioration, and welfare recipients, who, like the audience in Chicago, were beginning to tire of the continual forays of reformers into their lives. Despite these frustrations, one last full-dress effort at comprehensive welfare reform remained. Hoping to break the impasse, the Carter administration devoted considerable time and talent to the question. Some of the Carter welfare reformers, such as Michael Barth, a deputy assistant secretary of Health, Education, and Welfare, dated their welfare reform service from the days of the President's Commission on Income Maintenance. Barth reported to Assistant Secretary Henry Aaron, widely regarded as a brilliant economist, who had written on welfare at the Brookings Institution. Foreshadowing later difficulties, Aaron called his book *Why Is Welfare So Hard to Reform?* Aaron worked for HEW Secretary Joseph Califano, a tough and savvy Washington insider, who had served in Johnson's White House and played a key role in the creation of the Great Society. All in all, the Carter administration fielded a bright, experienced, and unsentimental team of welfare reformers.

Deeply interested in welfare reform and capable of plowing through complicated and lengthy memoranda on the subject, Carter nonetheless entrusted the details of welfare reform to Califano and to Ray Marshall, the Secretary of Labor. The cabinet secretaries negotiated a welfare reform plan. The process involved an awkward effort to combine the benefits of Califano's political sophistication, Aaron's expertise, and Marshall's desires to include a strong jobs component in the plan. The process consumed many computer runs, meetings, and cups of coffee, as once again a group of experts tried to solve the problems of social policy.

The group produced what its members believed was a new approach to welfare reform, a synthesis of the workfare and guaranteed income approaches. Called the President's Program for Better Jobs and Income, it relied on two tracks. Those along one track, the deserving poor, would receive a relatively high guaranteed income. Those along the other track, defined as people who were expected to work, would receive a lower guarantee and an opportunity to raise themselves above poverty by means of a guaranteed job. One variation of the program included an eight-week screening period during which the applicant received help in looking for a private-sector job. If he was unable to find a job, he received either a public service job or a government-subsidized job with a private employer.

Could the nation really manage to produce one and a half million jobs? Many within the administration entertained doubts. Charles Schultze, the chairman of the Council of Economic Advisers, advised Carter that the people holding the public service jobs might be engaged in make-work projects that were not much better than welfare. Carter believed the jobs could be found. He reasoned that, for the plan to succeed, three jobs would have to be created in Plains, Georgia, and found that goal not unreasonable. Whether he stopped to think about the 150,000 jobs that would be needed in New York City remained a matter of conjecture.

Carter announced his plan on August 6, 1977, almost exactly eight years after Nixon's announcement of FAP. The bill, like Nixon's, failed to pass, and its defeat signaled the end of the comprehensive reform effort.

By the 1980s, policymakers appeared content with Henry Aaron's advice that "simplicity is unachievable." Different folks deserved different strokes. Policymakers quietly abandoned the search for comprehensive reform.

The Frustrations of Welfare Reform

Rehabilitating the Poor

In the end, policymakers once again trotted out the idea of rehabilitating welfare recipients, and Congress geared up for another campaign, as though the entire history of welfare reform counted for
nothing. Welfare reform in the 1980s featured the story of Daniel
Moynihan and Ronald Reagan eyeing one another warily, moving
uneasily toward one another, and ending up in each other's laps.

When Ronald Reagan came to the White House in 1981, Robert
Carleson, his former state welfare director and now a presidential
advisor, handed David Stockman, the young director of the Office of
Management and Budget, a welfare plan and said, "Here is something
that has already been approved. All you have to do is plug it in. It's
like a cassette." Stockman "listened" to the cassette, liked what he
heard, and popped it into the budget. The changes included marginal
adjustments to AFDC, designed to help the truly poor and not aid
those capable of working. The changes looked small but, taken together, promised to save a billion dollars in 1982; as many as 400,000
people stood to lose their benefits.

Daniel Moynihan swallowed hard upon receiving news of the AFDC
cuts, and remarked that Reagan's budget went far toward erasing half
a century of social reform. Since Moynihan's days of working on the
FAP plan, he had served as Ambassador to India, Ambassador to the
United Nations, and been a professor of government at Harvard. In
1976, he won election to the Senate from the state of New York,
capping a remarkable career as an academic, diplomat, and politician.
In the Senate, he once again made welfare an area of special concern.
His appointment to the highly influential Committee on Finance,
which had charge of welfare and Social Security, reinforced this in-
terest, as did his new political goal of achieving fiscal relief for New
York City.

Once attacked by liberals as a racist for his report on the black
family and for a 1970 memorandum in which he suggested that the
"issue of race could benefit from a period of 'benign neglect,' " Moynihan now enjoyed a reputation as something of a prophet. His
thoughts on the black family appeared prescient. Neglected as a topic
of serious inquiry after 1965, the contemporary black family slowly
made its way back to the academic agenda. When William Julius
Wilson, a respected black sociologist from the University of Chicago,
checked on the matter, he found that things had only gotten worse
in the intervening years, much worse. If, as many had charged, Moynihan had overstated his case in 1965, it was difficult to do so in

1987, the year Wilson published *The Truly Disadvantaged.*

Wilson's calm, scholarly work recited chilling statistics. In 1965, the year of the Moynihan report, one-quarter of all black births occurred outside of marriage; by 1980, 57 percent of black births took place outside of marriage. When Moynihan wrote his report, women headed one-quarter of all black families; by 1980, this statistic had risen to 43 percent. Between 1960 and 1984, the proportion of non-white children in female-headed families tripled, going from 15 to 45 percent. Meanwhile, labor force participation rates among black women increased between 1940 and 1980, but the increase did not begin to match the increase in labor force participation among white women. Meanwhile, labor force participation rates of black men actually dropped, as did the percentage of black males who were employed.

Many blacks, according to Wilson, led disadvantaged lives in cities that contained relatively few people who were employed on a regular basis. White prejudice, once a matter of ethnicity, now, more than fifty years after large-scale immigration from Italy and Eastern Europe, became almost exclusively a matter of race. Without access to people with jobs, inner city black residents seldom discovered job opportunities or received recommendations for job openings. As job prospects declined, other prospects, such as welfare and the underground drug economy, became "increasingly relied on" and "seen as a way of life." Girls who became pregnant found few employed males to marry, exacerbating the trend toward illegitimacy.

Wilson saw the residents of the inner cities as "truly disadvantaged;" conservatives, rejuvenated by Ronald Reagan's emergence, regarded the residents of the inner cities as the victims of white benevolence. Conservative intellectuals, such as Charles Murray, asked what kept so many blacks chained to the inner city and its prospects of despair, and they decided the answer was welfare. Welfare, a distasteful but necessary form of social amelioration, in the liberal formulation, became a positive evil in the new conservative formulation.

In 1984, Charles Murray, a relatively obscure researcher in a relatively obscure think-tank, unable to move to a better tank because most were already well-stocked with liberals, published a book with a respectable press and a provocative title. *Losing Ground,* Murray's analysis of social policy from 1950 to 1980, caused a sensation, not seen on the borders of government and academia since the days when Michael Harrington, an equally obscure researcher with equally obscure connections, had published *The Other America* and made John F. Kennedy think about launching the War on Poverty.

Harrington's and Murray's books bracketed thirty years of intensive government anti-poverty and welfare reform efforts. Where Harrington helped launch the renaissance in government programs, Murray helped promote the counter reformation. Murray's book enabled the conservatives to claim the intellectual high ground by portraying government as the problem, not the solution.

Murray argued that not only had the social welfare system of the 1960s failed to meet its objectives but that, on balance, it had made people worse off. It had caused people to lose their will to work themselves out of poverty and had encouraged them to engage in destructive behavior. The Great Society had presented the poor not with a ladder of opportunity, but with a deep pit, a trap.

In 1985, Murray expanded on his ideas before the Joint Economic Committee. He began with the idea that jobs were available but public policy in the manner of the Great Society prevented people from taking them. True, the jobs paid poorly, but the welfare-induced family structure of the poor hindered them from banding together and pooling their wages. Afraid of leaving their subsidized housing in the slums, they hesitated to move where the jobs were in fact located—suburban Virginia, not downtown Washington, Westchester county, not the Bronx. When unemployed young people applied for a job, they often failed to get it because they lacked the language skills to be a sales clerk and the math skills to be a cashier. This erosion in skills reflected the influence of Title I of the Elementary and Secondary Education Act of 1965, which had stemmed from an "elite wisdom that decided it was wrong to compel students to absorb the habits and values of the majority middle class." And even if the person got the job and worked hard, he still needed to explain to his friends, "why he is willing to work for such chump change when they can make many times that, with much less effort and very little risk, dealing a little dope or fencing stolen goods."

For Murray and the new conservatives, the Great Society assumed the central role that the New Deal had played for the conservatives of the postwar era. Where conservatives once blamed FDR and the New Deal for the deterioration of America, they now saw Roosevelt as a traditional conservative doing his best to preserve America in a time of great economic stress. Lyndon Johnson became the preferred villain, as the man who perverted the New Deal programs. AFDC served as a good example. The new conservatives claimed that LBJ had changed this program in aid of worthy widows into a vehicle through which selfish people indulged their desire for children without marriage and forced taxpayers to pick up the check.

In the conservative view, the War on Poverty had acted as the agent that transformed AFDC from a worthy program to an engine of illegitimacy. It became the source of all evil for what two researchers from the Heritage Foundation called the "wooly thinking of the 1960s." It had helped people, but only by artificial means, such as boosting income by giving away welfare or raising employment by hiring people in make-work, makeshift public-sector jobs. Above all, the War on Poverty had made welfare a right, an absolute entitlement, that could not be rescinded for bad behavior and had, by breaking down the psychological barriers that kept people off the welfare rolls, increased welfare dependency.

Many conservatives criticized welfare programs by emphasizing the disparity between middle-class and lower-class women. More than half of all American women worked, including two-thirds of the women with children between six and thirteen. "Why on earth," asked Stuart Butler and Ann Kondratas of the Heritage Foundation, "should taxpaying working women, who only reluctantly leave their children to work, be taxed so that another group of women are able to stay home with theirs?"

In response to this conservative onslaught, liberals fell back on their complex views of public policy. For liberals, the problem of illegitimacy grew out of typically tangled causes. Careful statistical analysis, such as that performed by Harvard economist David Ellwood, suggested that between 1960 and 1984 the rise in the percentage of children living in female-headed families among whites paralleled the rise among blacks. The number of births to unmarried non-white women per 1,000 women of child-bearing age changed hardly at all between 1960 and 1984. However, births to married non-white women simply collapsed and, as a result, "out-of wedlock births as a percentage of all births to non-white women rose from 22 percent in 1960 to almost 50 percent in the 1980s." Ellwood also convincingly demonstrated that the rise in female-headed non-white families, contrary to the claims of Charles Murray, owed little to a rise in the welfare rate.

Other evidence, although hedged with the usual social science qualifications, argued that welfare was not the reason for black teenagers becoming pregnant. The very religious scruples, of which conservatives so approved, kept the girls from aborting their pregnancies. These same scruples, combined with the conservative resurgence in educational practice that took sex education out of the schools and into the ill-prepared home, also contributed to the girls' getting pregnant in the first place. "I thought," said one former welfare recipient and mother of several illegitimate children, "that if I ran to the bathroom after sex I wouldn't get pregnant." Once born, liberals asserted, babies, blameless for the mother's behavior, deserved support.

The complexities of liberalism played less well in the 1980s than they had in previous decades, nor had the liberals succeeded in any sense of the term. They failed to replace welfare with community action, a guaranteed income, or jobs. Manifestly, as the conservatives noted, the problem had gotten worse, despite all the money and computer time devoted to it.

Senator Moynihan knew all of that. He realized that to bring changes to welfare he would have to broker a deal between the conservatives and liberals. His chance came in February 1987 when the National Governors Association met in Washington and endorsed a welfare reform plan. "The leading innovations in this area have come from the states," announced the governors. Former governor and welfare reformer Ronald Reagan found this sentiment congenial and threw his support behind the governors' general approach to the problem.

However one characterized this approach, it stretched the truth to call it comprehensive reform. Instead, the approach represented a new version of workfare. Using the responsible rhetoric of private business, the governors called for a "binding, contractual agreement between the welfare recipient and the government," in which the rights and responsibilities of both parties were clearly delineated. The contract required welfare recipients, such as mothers with children three or older, to strive for self-sufficiency by engaging in training and looking for work. If they failed to meet their obligations, they lost their benefits, although not their children's benefits. The government promised to supply income, education and training, child care, medical care, and job placement to the recipient. If the government slipped, the recipient could settle back on welfare and enjoy a free ride.

The plan married Reagan's California approach to welfare and Jimmy Carter's vision of guaranteed jobs, with some distinctive twists. The governors put more emphasis on social services, such as day care, and on training as an investment than Reagan had done in his California plan. In contrast to Governor Reagan, the National Governors Association included in their plan government health insurance to cover former welfare recipients just starting out on a job. Unlike the Carter plan, the governors' proposal allowed the states considerable freedom to experiment with different approaches to providing welfare recipients with jobs.

The National Governors Association laid the groundwork for effective political compromise. Conservatives came to recognize the importance of social services such as medical care. Liberals came to understand that able-bodied people, even mothers of young children, must work.

Once the governors "jump-started" welfare reform, in the *Congressional Quarterly's* phrase, things moved quickly. Judged by the speed of previous welfare reforms, they positively raced. Months after the governors' meeting, four serious welfare reform proposals appeared in the House, all of which were in broad agreement on the need for workfare and disagreed only on how much to spend on it and whether or not to raise benefit levels. The House passed a final bill before Christmas 1987.

Meanwhile, Moynihan prepared a bill for the Senate that, as *Time* magazine reported, encouraged liberals to "recognize the importance of such conservative values as family, responsibility and work." These values, which had never been far from Moynihan's mind, served as the threads connecting the Moynihan report, FAP, and his current proposal. Moynihan's new bill represented his attempt to adapt his ideas to what *Time* called the "tough, tight-fisted" style of the Reagan era. The bill, like those of the governors and the House of Representatives, required welfare mothers with children over age three to participate in training and education programs. It also compelled absent fathers to support children by having payments deducted from their paychecks.

Here and there some liberal features appeared, such as the suggestion to provide nine months of medical benefits to working welfare mothers or to extend the AFDC–Unemployed Parents program, created by President Kennedy, to all of the states. For the most part, however, the bill emphasized using the creative energies of the states to put welfare mothers to work. "We took this approach," declared Moynihan, "not just to court the governors for their support, but because it is now the states—not the federal government—that seem to have the energy and creativity necessary to develop new, more productive approaches to public assistance." One could not, said Moynihan, "treat the teenagers of the 1980s as if they were widows of the 1930s," adding that, "You're never going to get a higher benefit until this is seen as a temporary program for people breaking out of dependency."

Once Moynihan's bill received the backing of the Senate Finance Committee, described by Spencer Rich of the *Washington Post* as "the traditional graveyard of overhaul proposals," it enjoyed clear sailing. Committee approval came on April 20, 1988, and the bill reached the floor very early in the summer and passed the Senate on June 16. President Reagan signed the Family Support Act of 1988 into law in October. The final version established comprehensive state education and training programs, transitional child care and medical assistance benefits, mandatory coverage for two-parent families for at least six months of each year, and stronger child support enforcement. With the passage of the act, the economists who worked in Washington gave the ball back to the social workers and manpower trainers who worked in the communities.

In the politicians' haste to do something about welfare in the period just preceding an election, they decided to ignore the historical record. The WIN program, for example, demonstrated the difficulties of putting welfare recipients to work and provided little reason to regard the new program with optimism. Moynihan himself expected that in the first few years of the program only ten percent of the families would become self-supporting, "but pretty soon, by the year 2,000, you have something to show for it."

Welfare and the Crisis of the Welfare State

The perpetual presence of people on the rolls defined welfare programs as failures and, particularly in hard economic times or times in which government deficits were sources of anxiety—that is to say, almost all the time—insured that the welfare system would be in a state of crisis.

Interactions between the Social Security and welfare programs heightened the feeling of crisis. In a sense, the former scooped the latter, picking off the easy cases and leaving welfare with the hard cases. Adding to welfare's burden, the measure of success for welfare became job placements and a diminution in the rolls, rather than, in the case of Social Security, retirement and an expansion in the number of beneficiaries. When welfare began, after all, the elderly constituted its major beneficiaries, but soon Social Security claimed those beneficiaries as its own and began mailing them retirement checks. When AFDC began, after all, widows and their children formed the largest group of beneficiaries, but Social Security soon claimed them as well. They, too, enjoyed the dignity of a crisp green check delivered to their doors. Only mothers and children without fathers remained as welfare recipients, and policymakers regarded a check in the mail as inappropriate for them. Welfare became the instrument of active rehabilitation, rather than passive payment.

This outcome ran directly counter to the original intentions of President Roosevelt, who wanted to get the federal government out of relief and who wanted to reserve federal welfare subsidies for the very young and the very old. Assumptions that had guided President Roosevelt, such as that neither women nor persons with disabilities

---

Welfare Restated, 1967–1988

belonged in the labor force, had crumbled. Similarly, policies that excluded blacks and other racial minorities, acceptable in Roosevelt's era, no longer were tenable. As a consequence, although Roosevelt never saw the welfare programs of the Social Security Act as a means of coping with the problems of illegitimacy, racial prejudice, and the decline of southern agriculture, they evolved into exactly that.

Policymakers devoted considerable creative energy to formulating alternatives to the traditional welfare system that reflected modern realities, but none of the alternatives worked. Providing suitable jobs, for example, constituted a difficult, perhaps impossible task, for which government at all levels was unequipped. Simply requiring people to work, perhaps accompanied by a guaranteed income—the single approach that might have been effective—proved impossible to implement. For one thing, work requirements violated rules of social compassion. The age of the poor house was over; government lacked the power to compel mothers caring for infants to work, nor could the government ban the birth of illegitimate children, for that violated liberals' sense of civil liberties and conservatives' sense of ethics.

For another thing, Social Security blocked the success of the guaranteed annual income. In a sense, Social Security represented a socially sanctioned form of a guaranteed annual income for the very young, the very old, labor force drop-outs caring for children, and disabled people. Criticism of a guaranteed income as reducing work effort thus became damning in part because the nation already paid a staggering amount to eliminate the work effort of Social Security beneficiaries and allow them to retire (except for the elderly over seventy who could work and still receive Social Security). The notion of a guaranteed annual income for a fifteen-year-old, illiterate, black girl pregnant with her second child ran into insurmountable political barriers, in part because Social Security had already creamed off the best welfare prospects.

It only made sense to offer a guaranteed income in the absence of other social benefits, and once the field became clogged with Social Security, Medicaid, food stamps, public housing, and the other remnants of past social policies, a guaranteed income became intellectually and politically impossible. A guaranteed annual income, no matter how it was constructed, created work disincentives, and the presence of the other programs made a difficult problem that much harder to solve.

These puzzles of social policy reflected the drive for a comprehensive solution to social problems that had come to characterize America since the 1960s. In the end, intelligent analysts concluded that a comprehensive solution could not be found and that the nation would have to blunder along with a jerry-rigged, piecemeal system of social benefits that overcompensated some, sapped the initiative of others, and failed even to reach still others.

Thus, the pattern of consensus in the 1950s and 1960s and of crisis in the 1970s and 1980s applied to welfare as well as to social insurance, although in a muted way. The welfare consensus proved to be weaker than that governing social insurance, and the welfare crisis stronger. The profound problems of welfare reform simply eluded solution. Instead, the romantic reform of the postwar consensus era that gave the nation a war on poverty and the rehabilitation approach to welfare ran its course and bequeathed a sense of crisis to the conservative era that followed.

★ ★ ★

III

The Mirage of National
Health Insurance

7   Medicare and Health Policy, 1935–1989

In April 1965, after the House of Representatives had passed the Medicare bill, the new program of health insurance for the elderly, Wilbur Cohen, the ebullient assistant secretary of Health, Education, and Welfare, received a package in the mail. Opening the package with his usual zest, Cohen discovered that it contained a gavel, sent to him by Representative John Dingell. The gavel, Dingell noted, was one of those used during the House debate on Medicare, over which Dingell had presided.

The symbolism immediately registered with Cohen. Dingell's father, also a congressman from Michigan, had tried without success to pass a national health insurance bill as part of the Social Security Board's cradle-to-grave protection plan. Now, more than twenty years later, the effort had proved successful, and the Speaker of the House had selected Dingell's son to preside over the historic session that marked the climax of a half-century of effort. Wrote Cohen in reply to Dingell, "I think it was both magnificent and proper that the Speaker should select you to preside over this auspicious occasion."

It was a momentous event for Cohen as well. Wilbur Cohen regarded the passage of Medicare as the legislative triumph of a long and productive life, yet Medicare, like the other programs of the New Deal and the Great Society, soon plunged into crisis. Asked in 1989 to describe Medicare, Deborah Steelman, who had worked for Presidents Reagan and Bush, said, "It's a mess." When Steelman spoke, she knew that without some action Medicare would go bankrupt by the turn of the century. She realized that as many as 37 million Americans had no health insurance and that the majority of the 9 million people who required long-term care had no insurance to pay for it. "There is not a person on the face of the earth who thinks this can be solved without a major restructuring of both public and private health-care systems," Steelman said.

In 1965, health insurance looked to be another pragmatic American triumph. Most people, according to the theory, received assistance from their employers that allowed them to pay their medical bills. In the meantime, they stored away money in the Social Security system that was used to buy a guaranteed health insurance policy that took effect upon retirement. Unlike other health insurance policies, this one could never be rescinded by the insurer, even for the very ill. The states provided health insurance for those, such as the people on welfare, who managed somehow to fall through the cracks. All in all, it amounted to a seamless system that represented our version of national health insurance.

The high costs of medical care soon undermined the system's coherence, and each of the major actors felt besieged. People without health insurance hoped that their family members would not become sick. When members of such a family did, in fact, become ill and entered a hospital, they threw themselves on the hospital's mercy. Hospitals complained loudly and publicly about the burden of providing uncompensated care. The federal government scrambled unsuccessfully to cover the rising costs of Medicare. The states began to find Medicaid, their end of the system, an intolerable burden. One official of the National Governors Association said in 1989, "The 'feds' have been living on their credit card for years. Now, by mandating to us the things that they can't afford, they're trying to use ours." Private employers protested that health care costs were cutting into their profits and, some claimed, making it more difficult to compete against the Japanese. A spokesman for the National Association of Manufacturers observed in 1989 that, "health care is the issue of the hour, the No. 1 concern of our members." Lee Iacocca, the charismatic Chrysler salesman, citing figures that showed his company spent $600 per car on health care or nearly three times what the Japanese companies spent, said, "American industry cannot compete effectively with the rest of the world unless something is done about the great imbalance between health care costs in the U.S. and the national health care systems in virtually every other country."

The First National Health Insurance System

The story of national health insurance, like that of Social Security and welfare, went back to the Social Security Act itself. When President

Roosevelt authorized the Committee on Economic Security to begin its work, health insurance already figured prominently in the discussion. At the time, health insurance, as the term was understood, included the income a person lost during illness (disability insurance) as well as the costs of treating the illness (health insurance). If anything, disability income mattered more then health care, since an extended period of disability might wipe out a family's savings.

The cost of treatment, although an important risk that all families faced, involved paying a few bills, and in the 1920s, the overwhelming majority of Americans, rich or poor, paid the bills out of their own pockets. Doctors helped poorer families by adjusting their fees along a "sliding scale," so that a person disbursed only what he could afford. Hospitals, also, accepted a number of charity patients and offered different accommodations to the rich and the poor. Wealthier people enjoyed a room of their own; poorer people shared a room with others.

By the 1930s, reflecting the convergence of economic, scientific, and cultural forces, the costs of medical care had emerged as an important source of financial insecurity. In 1934, experts, using data from the late 1920s, estimated that a family earning less than $1200 still spent $43 or 5.2 percent of its income on medical services. Such costs loomed large in the Depression era. Furthermore, postponing these costs carried serious consequences, since neglecting health care, according to the conventional wisdom, meant a serious deterioration in a person's productivity and well-being. New photo magazines, like *Life*, portraying medicine as a source of scientific progress and of hope against dread disease, reinforced this positive image of health care. Increasingly, then, health care became something desirable; and to be denied access to it amounted to social deprivation.

President Roosevelt and Edwin Witte, staff director of the Committee on Economic Security, invited two public health experts, both of whom had worked on an earlier and well-publicized study on the costs of medical care, to draft health care proposals for the committee. These experts, Edgar Sydenstricker and I. S. Falk, employees of the Milbank Memorial Fund, eagerly obliged. In September 1934, they produced preliminary suggestions for an American health and disability program that could be folded into the Social Security legislation.

Falk and Sydenstricker made much of foreign precedent. Other countries included protection against disability and ill health as part of their national social insurance programs, and America should do the same. The "progressive nations" had experimented with health insurance, and the foreign programs had met with great success.

Medicare and Health Policy, 1935–1989

Without national health insurance and without substantial commercial insurance protection, America lagged behind the world. We had never managed to pool the costs of ill health broadly enough to keep individual costs within manageable limits.

If Americans wished to emulate this foreign success, they needed to budget the costs of medical care on a group basis, so that each family would carry an average rather than an uncertain risk. Under the old system, a healthy family paid nothing because its members never saw the doctor or went to the hospital; an unhealthy family faced catastrophic costs. Falk and Sydenstricker, who wanted to even out this burden, believed that if enough people participated, the cost to each family would be well within a family's means. That meant that neither the government nor employers had to make special contributions to national health insurance, because the costs of insurance would be "substantially within people's means even if they had to pay all of the costs themselves."

Health insurance, which would be greeted as a "great benefaction," could therefore be America's first form of social insurance. Other forms of social insurance, such as unemployment compensation and old-age insurance, required time consuming preparation periods. In old-age insurance, for example, the government needed to gather large financial reserves over a period of five years before pensions could be paid. Nothing similar applied to health insurance; Falk and Sydenstricker believed that it could be put into operation within 90 days. After all, the health care system already existed. Falk and Sydenstricker simply proposed to make it easier for people to pay the bills.

Even Falk and Sydenstricker realized, however, that things were not quite so simple. If they had been, national health insurance would have become a legacy of the New Deal. Instead, national health insurance stalled, in part because an acceptable national system of health care provision did not yet exist. In the 1930s, some people, particularly those in rural areas, could not go to a general hospital because there was none in their community. As late as 1945, a Senate subcommittee found that 40 percent of the counties in the United States lacked hospital facilities, and many of these also suffered from a shortage of physicians.

In addition, Falk and Sydenstricker's suggestions to alter the health care financing system aroused the suspicions of the doctors who provided the care. Doctors, the beneficiaries of so much acclaim from the media, recognized that the line between shoring up the present system and creating a new system was a fine one. Some doctors thought that national health insurance would change the system for the worse.

The Mirage of National Health Insurance

Taken together, these things raised sufficient doubts to postpone national health insurance. Falk and Sydenstricker learned late in 1934 that health insurance would not be included in the Social Security bill that the Roosevelt administration would submit to Congress. As the Social Security Act encountered delays in passage, the administration proved more and more reluctant to submit a separate health insurance bill, and decided to wait until after the 1936 election. Although Senator Wagner finally introduced a health and disability bill in 1939, one that relied on federal grants to the states, the bill became stalled in committee and never received serious consideration.

By the next year, conditions had changed so completely that the Roosevelt Administration began to rethink its approach to health and disability legislation. The passage of the Social Security Act, the race with welfare, and the end of the Depression altered the politics of national health insurance. Instead of a public, centralized approach to health care finance, the nation ended up choosing a private, community-based approach.

Changing styles of bureaucratic politics played an important role in the demise of national health insurance. In 1935, Congress authorized two types of social insurance laws. Old-age insurance, the first type, depended on centralized, federal administration; unemployment compensation, the second type, relied on decentralized, state administration. But by the early 1940s, the Social Security bureaucrats grew dissatisfied with this approach and wanted to substitute a purely federal system for the prevailing mixed system. As a consequence, they floated the grand Wagner-Murray-Dingell scheme of 1943, complete with federal health, permanent disability, unemployment, and temporary disability insurance.

As the bureaucratic paradigm for national health insurance shifted, national health insurance suddenly became more complicated and less appealing. Group budgeting, the old idea for national health insurance, gave way to extending the Social Security system, the new idea for national health insurance. The new association between national health insurance and old-age insurance weakened the health insurance cause. Social Security remained trapped in its unpromising race with welfare. Congress, not yet ready to increase Social Security benefits, hardly felt predisposed to approve a national health insurance program funded through the Social Security system. Simply put, government-financed national health insurance got nowhere in the 1940s, and Falk and Sydenstricker's simple idea of "group budgeting," charging everyone the average cost of care, surfaced in the private rather than the public sector.

In the 1940s, a revolution in health care finance occurred without the direct intervention of the federal government. Third-party payment of medical bills became the norm, rather than the exception. In part, the revolution reflected the fact that, with the Depression over, more people could afford to purchase private health insurance, which increasingly became available as one of the fringe benefits that Americans earned on the job.

Blue Cross plans led the way. These community-based and locally controlled "assurance" plans enabled Americans to prepay their hospital bills through level, predictable "premiums." A certain sum of money bought a certain number of days in the hospital. Begun at the end of the 1920s, the plans contained more than a million members by the end of the 1930s. By 1951, membership in the plans had skyrocketed to 37.4 million people. By then, more than half of the patients in hospitals entered with some form of hospital insurance, compared with only 9 percent in 1940.

By 1951, as well, private insurance to pay doctors' bills reached more than 40 million people. The great majority of the policies intruded on the private practice of medicine in the gentlest possible manner. An individual could go to any doctor, pay the bill, and then send the bill to the insurance company, which determined whether the visit was reimbursable and, if it was, sent the individual a check to cover some of the expense.

Through these forms of insurance coverage, Falk and Sydenstricker's vision of group budgeting came to be realized. Employees of a plant or industry and their families, not the citizens of an entire state or the whole nation, formed the groups that together comprised a national system of health insurance. If the system left wide gaps in coverage, it nonetheless represented a health care financing scheme, the very presence of which made a federal plan, tied to the politically unpopular Social Security system, less necessary to have and more difficult to enact.

Temporary Disability Insurance

The related field of disability insurance followed a similar pattern in the 1930s and 1940s. Proposals for a national, federal plan resulted instead in a state and privately administered system with limited coverage.

Initially, the very size of the problem caused people to hesitate. With the need for income so desperate during the Depression, people thought twice about pensions that were payable on the basis of physical disability. They worried that the government would not be able to keep the costs within manageable limits and feared that the permanently unemployed would use disability as a convenient ticket out of the labor force.

With policymakers hesitant to initiate a disability insurance program, two alternatives surfaced. Since many disabled people were over sixty-five, old-age insurance served as an ersatz form of permanent disability insurance. For someone still working, policymakers proposed a temporary disability program or "sick pay." If a worker became ill and left work for up to six months, temporary disability insurance, an old form of social benefit that dated from the German social insurance program of the 1880s, would protect him against the loss of some of his income. In America, with the exception of compensation for temporary disability that resulted from a work injury, such a program did not yet exist.

As happened with health insurance, bureaucratic politics made a difference. In 1943, federal bureaucrats hoped to make temporary disability insurance part of the grand federal cradle-to-grave social insurance system, but their hopes met with disappointment. States and private companies preempted the federal government. Rhode Island passed a temporary disability law in 1942; by the end of the decade, five states administered temporary disability laws. Employers in most states did not need a state law to compel them to offer temporary disability insurance. Instead, temporary disability became another of the fringe benefits that employers provided to their employees.

The state laws and the private plans inhibited the Social Security Board's efforts to initiate a federal temporary disability program as part of the proposed cradle-to-grave coverage. In 1949, Wilbur Mills, already an influential member of the House Committee on Ways and Means, asked why Congress should bother with a federal law when the states were experimenting with cash sickness benefits. Insurance executives opposed federal temporary disability insurance because it would leave, in the words of one Equitable Life Assurance official, no room for the "preservation of numerous voluntary plans." A personnel director of a large southern textile firm claimed in 1949 that temporary disability plans already covered 32,000,000 employees.

States that passed temporary disability laws took pains not to interfere with voluntary, private plans. In New Jersey, for example, employers, who were required to provide temporary disability insurance, could elect to use a state-run insurance system or a private plan, such as the Equitable might sell. In New York, the director of the temporary disability insurance program took as her objective, "to disturb as little as possible the thousands of welfare plans which have already been developed and that now afford disability benefits for at least 60 percent of all employees in New York State." She wanted to guard against "statism."

As the cases of health insurance and temporary disability insurance illustrated, America developed a welfare state based in large part on indirect government subsidies—through tax policy—of private social benefits. This strategy fit the more general American model for social policy: the use of tax policy to manage the economy and encourage socially beneficial yet privately controlled behavior.

Government and the Medical Infrastructure

Even beyond the use of tax policy, however, it would be a mistake to assume that government played no role in the nation's postwar health policy. Health care operated less as a private than as a community concern. Hospitals tended to be community-based, not-for-profit institutions. The health insurance industry existed within a highly regulated environment in which the states laid down the rules, such as the level of financial reserves that companies were required to have on hand to pay claims.

Further, the Blue Cross programs, which constituted the most important mechanism for financing hospital care during the 1930s and 1940s, resembled hospitals in being nonprofit and community based. These programs marketed themselves as alternatives to traditional private insurance, in part because they charged a "universal" rate, applicable to all, rather than a rate that varied with a company's or an individual's claims experience. In recognition of Blue Cross's special community service, the states passed laws exempting Blue Cross plans from insurance regulations.

For all of government's interest in health care, *federal* health policy remained a problematic matter. Education provided the best analogy. As in the field of education, where a community's preferences concerning how to teach about sensitive matters such as evolution or religion conferred a certain sanctity upon them that Congress seldom challenged, local discretion left little room for a federal health policy. Neither Congress nor the federal government wished to prescribe a regimen of medical treatment, any more than it wanted to outline a science curriculum.

In both cases, however, although the details were left with local and professional communities, people who agreed that education and health care represented something of value sought unobtrusive ways of spending federal money on them. Both education and health represented good investments in the nation's future. Furthermore, economic considerations dictated that government, rather than individual entrepreneurs, should undertake the investment, because the benefits, and hence the true profits, of a good hospital or school spilled over into the entire community.

The notion of investing in the health care system through the construction of facilities and the creation of useful knowledge served as the rationale for federal health policy in the 1940s. Delicately asserting the federal government's role as the creator of a medical infrastructure, federal bureaucrats disavowed any intention to control either the financing or the provision of actual care.

On August 13, 1946, President Harry Truman signed into law the Hospital Survey and Construction Act. The law initiated a program of federal grants to be used for surveying a state's needs for more hospitals and for building the hospitals themselves. An earlier version of a national hospital bill, introduced in 1940, had called for direct federal funding of hospital construction and federal ownership of the hospitals. The successful version was endorsed by a wide coalition of political interests stretching from the Chamber of Commerce and the American Medical Association on the right to labor unions and the Social Security bureaucracy on the left. It put local authorities firmly in charge of local hospitals.

The congressional committee considering the legislation stressed the need for more hospitals, as if the expansion of modern facilities would in itself solve the problems of gaining access to medical care. According to the committee, hospitals were crucial to the development of adequate medical care, since advances in medical science had made medicine "increasingly more technical and complex, requiring the best modern facilities and equipment for its successful practice." And without good hospitals, the committee stressed, a community could not be expected to attract good doctors. As a consequence, wealthier metropolitan areas were being better served than poorer rural areas. The congressional committee believed that the federal government should supply help to the rural areas. The need was so pressing, according to the committee, that organizations "traditionally opposed to requesting federal assistance in working out their problems expressed the view that federal assistance is indispensable."

Conferring federal largess on the hospital, rather than on the doctors who practiced in the hospital, proved to be a shrewd political choice. Over the course of a century, the hospital had undergone an amazing transformation. In the middle of the nineteenth century, the hospital functioned as a welfare institution, drawing its patients from the poor people who had few roots in the community. Being a hospital patient meant taking charity. In 1870, Boston's Massachusetts General

Hospital served an average of 120 patients at any one time, 89 of whom qualified as free or charity patients. What happened inside the hospital differed considerably from the workings of a modern hospital. Far from the high-technology events of today, hospital births provided an inferior alternative to giving birth at home, and many babies born in hospitals were illegitimate. Most doctors, whatever their specialty, kept track of their patients at home. Little that was done in the hospital could not be duplicated with the tools commonly found in the kitchen.

At the end of the nineteenth century, hospitals began to resemble modern hospitals. They became theaters for the performance of surgery. As hospitals began to take care of sick people rather than dependent people, the economic status of their clientele rose. By 1920, more than half of the typical hospital's income came from private patients, rather than from private donors. Within the hospital, accommodations improved. No longer a place with wards full of patients who were expected to follow strict rules dedicated to moral uplift, such as not playing cards, the hospital became filled with private and semi-private rooms.

As hospitals grew in stature, creating more of them became a national priority. The modern hospital, no longer an asylum, was too expensive to be maintained by patients' fees alone. Hence, the Hospital Survey and Construction Act provided a welcome source of funds for a widely acclaimed institution. The funds benefited medicine without presuming to dictate the terms of medical practice. Depending on a person's political point of view, money for hospital construction marked the final solution to health care problems or an incremental step toward national health insurance. The act consequently encountered few political difficulties, even at a time when national health insurance was being contested along deep partisan lines.

Funds for medical research, another feature of the federal government's investment in medicine, also began to flow in earnest in 1946. The National Mental Health Act exemplified the general phenomenon. Mental health hospitals, unlike general hospitals, remained asylums well into this century. In Massachusetts during the 1930s, as historian Gerald Grob has noted, long-term patients, many of whom were elderly, filled nearly 80 percent of the available mental health beds. In 1940 public mental health hospitals, which cared for nearly 98 percent of all institutionalized patients, had a resident population of 410,000. "Simply put," writes Grob, "mental hospitals provided custodial long-term care for a variety of dependent persons who were unable to survive without assistance."

Psychiatrists, trained in medicine, rebelled against this setting for their specialty. They, like their fellow doctors, wanted to be seen as skilled practitioners who *cured* patients, rather than as people who took custody of chronic invalids. They preferred to work in the dignified surroundings of community or university hospitals, rather than within the dismal confines of state mental health asylums.

Dr. Robert Felix, of the Public Health Service, drafted a bill for a national mental health program. A shrewd practitioner of medical politics, Felix enlisted the support of Mary Switzer, a key assistant to the person who would today be called the secretary of Health and Human Services, the support of the Menninger brothers of Topeka, Kansas, and of Mary Lasker, a wealthy layperson interested in medical research. His preparation paid important dividends. When J. Percy Priest, a Tennessee congressman, expressed an interest in mental health legislation, Switzer handed him a completed draft for a bill. Hearings went quickly, and the bill became law on July 3, 1946.

The law had three basic purposes: to provide support for mental health research; to establish grants to train psychiatrists; to make available support for mental health clinics and treatment centers. It specified that financial aid be for these modern centers, rather than the old system of state mental health hospitals.

Taken as a whole, the federal government's commitment to the cause of medical research in the postwar era was impressive. The National Institutes of Health (NIH), the center of the medical research bureaucracy and the chief dispenser of funds for medical research, saw its budget go from $7 million in fiscal year 1947 to $70 million in the first year of Dwight Eisenhower's presidency. In some of those years, Congress granted the NIH more money than it had officially requested.

The commitment to medical facilities and research reflected a postwar sense of optimism that diseases could be cured, and it enabled America to approach the 1950s with a broad policy on health care that resembled the Social Security program in its pragmatic mix of public and private elements. One could not neatly categorize governmental and nongovernmental responsibilities, yet such a categorization hardly seemed to matter. The American political system had once again taken a problem considered to have broad ideological overtones, had compromised the differences, and had produced a workable, if not exactly coherent, solution.

The sensible solution offered many people the chance to purchase health insurance. Reasonably priced health insurance in turn purchased what was perceived as constantly improving health care. Medicine got better and better, the theory went, in part because of the progress that was inherent in science and in part because of increasing federal investment in medical research and facilities. Health care therefore fit the mid-century American consensus in social welfare policy neatly.

Permanent Disability Insurance

Where some saw progress, others perceived significant gaps. Many people had health insurance, for example, but the elderly still encountered significant problems. Because they were no longer working, they had no group in which to pool the costs of their medical care, which was, in any event, more costly than that received by younger people. One could patch together solutions, such as collectively bargained health care for retirees, but any such patchwork plans tended to leave many of the elderly uncovered.

In 1951, Wilbur Cohen, then an assistant to the head of the Social Security Board, got an idea that met with an immediately favorable response. He thought it might be possible to use one element of the social welfare consensus, the new-found popularity of old-age insurance, to alter another element of the consensus, the private system of health care finance. In a memo to the Federal Security Administration, he proposed establishment of health insurance for Social Security beneficiaries. Previous plans, such as the Wagner-Murray-Dingell bill of 1943, had looked toward national health insurance for people of all ages. Now, Cohen favored health insurance only for the elderly people getting Social Security benefits. The idea could be sold to Congress as an extension of Social Security rather than as a plan to reorganize the health care finance system. Oscar Ewing, the head of the Federal Security Agency, became excited about the idea as soon as he read the memo. Medicare was launched.

Before Congress could pass Medicare, however, it needed to dispose of disability insurance, another important piece of Social Security business. Although federal temporary disability insurance was a lost cause, insurance for permanent disability, defined as a person's inability to work for the rest of his life due to physical causes, remained politically viable. It came before Medicare on the agenda in part because Congress had already spent a great deal of time on it. The Social Security advisory council that met in 1948 had proposed a limited program of permanent disability insurance. The advisory council's plan received the endorsement of the House Committee on Ways and Means and passed the House of Representatives but then was killed by the Senate Committee on Finance.

Permanent disability insurance encountered political problems in

The Mirage of National Health Insurance

the crossfire of the national health insurance debate. Between the middle and the end of the 1940s, the American Medical Association began a course of strict opposition to federal disability legislation. The AMA reasoned that permanent disability insurance would serve as the entering wedge for national health insurance. Once the government hired doctors to decide if a person was disabled, it was only a matter of time before the government would ask doctors to participate in a national health insurance program, and in no time doctors would become thoroughly regimented government employees. Far better, representatives of the AMA believed, to limit disability protection to the truly needy who could be closely monitored by local authorities. Welfare was superior to social insurance for this purpose. Congress, wary of taking on the doctors and the insurance industry as well, shied away from disability insurance.

The campaign for permanent disability insurance involved constant bureaucratic reassurances to congressmen that disability would not upset the consensus on which social welfare policy rested. Most people retired at age sixty-five. Those who became disabled before that age watched passively as their Social Security benefits dwindled. If they managed to reach 65, they received a pittance or, worse, nothing at all. Most fell back on the demeaning alternative of welfare. The country, with its affluent economy and its well-stocked Social Security trust funds, could afford to do better. Congress should therefore take the next modest step in Social Security and allow the disabled, those who could prove that they were not fit to work anymore, the humane choice of early retirement.

When, in 1956, Social Security's popularity became too much for Congress to resist and the doctors to oppose, permanent disability insurance became law. The program consisted of federal financing, through the Social Security payroll tax, and state administration.

A person applying for disability benefits followed a slightly different course than did an applicant for old-age benefits. The disability application started just like any other Social Security request. A person went to a local office, explained the situation, and requested the forms to apply for disability benefits. The local Social Security officer checked to see that the person had worked for enough time in the right places to qualify for benefits. But the local officer made no attempt to determine if the person was truly disabled, that is, "unable to engage in substantial gainful activity." That determination came from a state-run office, often part of the state's vocational rehabilitation program, that specialized in gathering medical and vocational evidence and deciding whether a person met the disability definition.

With the passage of disability insurance in 1956, the vocational rehabilitation programs acquired the important responsibility of making disability determinations for the Social Security Administration. The theory that motivated this change depended on political and psychological reassurances to doctors, conservative congressmen, and the Eisenhower administration. On the political level, state control of disability decisions took some of the menace from the extension of the welfare state to cover disability. States could be expected to exercise more caution than the federal government in declaring someone eligible for a disability pension.

On the psychological level, the decision to let the states administer the disability insurance program introduced a positive note into a negative program. Rather than a program for labor force drop-outs, disability insurance became a means of putting disability applicants in touch with the rehabilitation counselors. Some people, beyond salvation, would be pensioned off, allowed to retire. Other people would be directed to the vocational rehabilitation program, told of their potential, and placed in a program of training, advice, and medical care. Such people would rethink their desire to retire. Newly energized, they would decide against cashing in their working lives and opt instead for the therapeutic course of working.

Together, political, psychological, and bureaucratic tangles created a social policy snafu. The completed legislation restricted benefits to people fifty or older and that limited the effectiveness of the rehabilitation approach. State counselors achieved little success rehabilitating people who were already fifty or older, suffering from a physical impairment, and interested enough in retirement to apply for disability benefits. As a consequence, this rehabilitation link in social policy, just like the ones in the welfare programs, never took hold, leaving the country with an anomalous bureaucratic structure in which the states worked under contract to the federal government and made disability determinations.

Toward Medicare

Social Security Administration officials, who had pushed for the passage of disability insurance and had danced in the aisles of the Senate observers gallery when the measure finally passed, cared little about rehabilitation. They continued to work for the passage of Medicare. Once again, they made compromises for political reasons, and once again the compromises worked, bringing political success in 1965. As with disability policy, however, the compromises produced a complicated piece of legislation that led to more social policy snafus.

Not surprisingly, the first serious Medicare bill appeared the year

The Mirage of National Health Insurance

after the passage of disability insurance. Introduced by Rhode Island Congressman Aime Forand, a junior member of the House Ways and Means Committee, it included hospitalization, surgical, and convalescent benefits.

A small group of Social Security insiders wrote the Forand bill. Important members included Cohen, now a professor at the University of Michigan, I. S. Falk, part of the 1934 team that had produced the first Social Security health proposal and now teaching at Yale, Robert Ball, still a key Social Security official, and Nelson Cruikshank. A gentle man but one passionately devoted to the social insurance cause, Cruikshank, who worked for organized labor, enjoyed the confidence of George Meany, the head of the AFL-CIO.

These individuals continued to press the logic of the social insurance approach. A small donation for every worker bought a large program. For only 0.5 percent of covered payroll, as the jargon went, one could initiate a program containing 60 days of hospitalization, protection against the doctors' bills after surgery, and 60 days of nursing home care. That meant someone already paying Social Security could get medical coverage at retirement for a few dollars more each year.

The logic of collective action, although seductive, contained obvious political and more subtle ideological problems. On the purely political level, the doctors resisted national health insurance, even when limited to the elderly, as the precursor to insurance covering people of all ages. The expansion of disability insurance to include benefits for the dependents of the disabled (1958) and benefits for disabled people of all ages (1960) added substance to the doctors' fears. Social Security officials tried to calm the doctors by limiting benefits, in the style of Blue Cross plans, to hospitalization. Although some, who owed their first allegiance to health insurance rather than to Social Security, objected, others saw the political attractiveness of excluding doctors' fees. In this manner, politics shaped the contours of the Medicare proposal.

The chief political strategy remained one of using the popularity of Social Security to gain passage of Medicare, even though this strategy shaded the truth. As nearly everyone realized, Medicare differed from old-age insurance. In old-age insurance, officials made an elaborate effort to create the illusion that a person saved for his retirement. In Medicare, this illusion could not be sustained. Instead, it was obvious that current workers paid the medical bills of current retirees. After all, plans called for paying Medicare benefits immediately rather than waiting to build up a trust fund. That meant that those who were already old would receive Medicare for free.

Nor could the relationship between the money collected and the money spent be predicted with the same accuracy as in old-age insurance. In old-age insurance, it was demography, the number of older people in the population, that mattered most; and, although one could not be certain about this number, one could at least make educated guesses. In health insurance, economics, the cost of medical services, mattered more than did the number of people eligible for services; and, although one could make cost estimates, the accuracy of these estimates remained questionable.

None of these problems halted the Medicare movement. The passage of disability insurance, with its many internal compromises, convinced Cohen, Ball, and the others of their political prowess. Accordingly, they bargained their way toward the Medicare program, justifying such compromises as excluding doctors' bills from the program and limiting the program to retired Social Security beneficiaries. They believed that today's inadequacies become the subjects of tomorrow's legislation.

This attitude gave the advocates of Medicare a flexibility that the doctors lacked. The doctors opposed almost all federal health insurance legislation as the start of national health insurance. The Medicare advocates appeared willing to accommodate the doctors by agreeing to compromise legislation.

Meanwhile, the pressure for Medicare continued to build, breaking out in the open during 1960. Congress conducted hearings in which the lack of health care was presented as a unique problem of the elderly, neatly separating measures for the elderly from the more general and ideological battle over what the American Medical Association called "socialized" medicine. John F. Kennedy, running for president and wishing to associate himself with Presidents Roosevelt and Truman in domestic affairs, openly endorsed Medicare. In a neat bit of symbolic politics, he celebrated the twenty-fifth anniversary of the Social Security Act with a speech at Hyde Park, the shrine dedicated to Franklin Roosevelt. Within sight of Franklin Roosevelt's grave, in front of thousands of people, Kennedy ended a longstanding feud with Eleanor Roosevelt, lauded Social Security, and endorsed Medicare. It was a powerful conjunction of political images.

The Republicans knew that they needed a counterproposal and so they, too, came up with a health insurance plan, for Richard Nixon to use in 1960. Arthur Flemming, the Eisenhower administration's liberal but loyal secretary of Health, Education, and Welfare, produced a scheme that included 180 days of hospitalization and covered most other medical expenses. This plan differed from social insurance, as the term was understood at the time, because the elderly themselves, rather than current workers, would pay for it, because the states and private companies would administer it, and because it would involve a "means" test that resulted in different treatment of the rich and the poor.

The Kerr-Mills Proposal

Wilbur Mills, the chairman of the House Committee on Ways and Means, who opposed Medicare as too costly and the Republican plan on political grounds, sought his own alternative. With the help of Senator Robert Kerr, a powerful Oklahoma legislator who exercised considerable influence over the Senate Finance Committee, Mills put together another health insurance plan for the elderly. This one followed a welfare or public assistance format. Federal grants enabled states to pay for the medical care of elderly welfare recipients or for the care of elderly persons too poor to pay their own medical bills but too rich to qualify for welfare. States, many of which already devoted part of their welfare budget to funding medical care, received the freedom to devise their own medical care arrangements.

The Kerr-Mills proposals tested the willingness of the Medicare advocates to compromise. For some, who regarded welfare as anathema, the Kerr-Mills program deserved no more consideration than did the Republican program. Robert Ball, writing to a liberal congressman, termed any public assistance program "unsatisfactory" because it involved the "humiliation of a means test." Social insurance, as contrasted with public assistance in Ball's mind, "supports the individual's self-reliance and independence and helps to prevent poverty." That, to people like Ball, defined the key distinction: preventing poverty as in social insurance, or waiting for it to occur, as in public assistance.

For others in the coalition, Kerr-Mills deserved support not because it was the solution to the health insurance problem but because it was a step toward the solution. Some people saw Kerr-Mills as a realistic alternative to Medicare and hence a stumbling block to Medicare's adoption. Other people viewed Kerr-Mills more as just another piece of health legislation and less as an alternative to Medicare. Kerr-Mills, they thought, would not deter and might even aid in the battle for Medicare and the fight for national health insurance that lay beyond that. Wilbur Cohen, for one, lent Mills and Kerr his support and his technical expertise in drafting the legislation.

Cohen proved quite astute. Kerr-Mills did little to impede and much to help the passage of Medicare. Once adopted, the Kerr-Mills program demonstrated the inconsistency of state approaches to health care finance and the inability of many states to handle the problem.

Events in Texas illustrated the inadequacy of state efforts. In 1961, responding to popular interest and political pressure, Texas began a formal medical program for elderly people on welfare. Texas had a population of nearly 10.5 million people, about 8 percent of whom were over sixty-five. In 1964, two-thirds of the aged collected Social Security benefits and about one-third were on the welfare rolls, receiving an average payment of $58 a month.

The state never joined the Kerr-Mills program; it simply took advantage of other federal grants and of its own resources and used those resources to start a hospital insurance program. If an elderly person receiving welfare went into the hospital, the state would pay $10 a day for 15 days and $6 a day beginning on the 16th day. Under this arrangement, poor elderly patients tended to get released from the hospital sooner than other elderly patients, even sooner than the elderly on welfare in other states. Hospitals, although hardly excited about this rate of reimbursement, knew they would be unable to collect much in the way of additional fees from the patients themselves.

In 1963, the conservative Texas legislature decided to take another step toward granting the elderly access to health care. It enacted a law that allowed private health insurance companies to join together and market a collective health insurance plan for aged Texans. Private carriers, under pressure to demonstrate that they could handle this market, came up with a surgical insurance policy, costing $9 a month, and a major medical plan, priced at $10 a month. Only about 45,000 people signed up for the plans, less than 6 percent of the eligible population. One reason, surely, was that the combined cost of the two plans, $228 a year, was about one-third of a single elderly person's income. The Texas case demonstrated the difficulties of successfully marketing a private health insurance plan for the elderly.

Case studies of this type became important pieces of propaganda in the hands of the Medicare proponents. Other pieces of evidence came from states that did pass Kerr-Mills programs or from states that tried and failed to pass such programs. Only thirty-six states managed to pass a Kerr-Mills program by 1963. Proposals failed in Arizona, Colorado, Ohio, Montana, and Rhode Island. Governors in Indiana and Missouri vetoed programs already passed by their legislatures. Passage of the Nevada program hinged on a state referendum that the voters rejected. These bits of evidence demonstrated how inconsistent the programs were from state to state and how capriciously the states handled the problem.

The Final Campaign

If the states were not the answer to health care for the elderly, then perhaps the federal government would administer a program, as many had hoped for nearly twenty years. The election of President Kennedy in 1960 advanced the Medicare cause, because it meant that the Medicare advocates, working in official capacities, could come out of the closet and openly advocate the measure that the Eisenhower administration had not officially endorsed. Kennedy's election also brought Wilbur Cohen back from Ann Arbor to Washington to help engineer the campaign.

Kennedy's thin victory, however, provided the administration with no particular mandate for Medicare. In general, the administration's domestic initiatives faced considerable scrutiny from a Congress that was concerned, as it had been since the end of World War II, with protecting state's rights and that feared the use of federal power to promote civil rights legislation. Kennedy himself, in common with Truman and Eisenhower, staked his reputation on international, rather than domestic affairs.

Congressional proprietors of Social Security, such as Wilbur Mills, continued to resist Medicare, and without Mills's approval, there would be no Medicare program. Mills's misgivings stemmed as much from his desire to preserve the Social Security program as from any fundamental streak of conservatism. Although Wilbur Cohen and Robert Ball tried to reassure Mills that Medicare, like disability insurance, was only a modest and necessary extension of Social Security, Mills balked. He worried that health insurance would serve as the vehicle to bring general revenues into the program and that it would require constant raises in Social Security taxes. No longer would Congress be able to vote handsome increases in Social Security benefits every two years and continue to reap the financial bonanza of postwar recovery. Instead, Congress would constantly need to feed the Medicare program with more funds, like parking a car at a twenty minute meter and leaving it there.

As the administration wooed Wilbur Mills, it reduced its bill to the bare essentials, in keeping with the standard procedure that produced the Medicare bill in the first place. The bill, like its predecessors, limited its benefits to the elderly and, at least for purposes of public discussion, conceded groups other than the elderly to the private sector and the health care consensus. "The federal government," said

HEW Secretary Anthony Celebrezze, reassuring one medical doctor, "need not get involved in this area."

A series of other concessions shaped the Medicare bill. It covered hospital bills but not doctors' bills because the administration could work with the American Hospital Association but not with the American Medical Association and because paying physicians represented another area in which, as Celebrezze might have put it, the government need not get involved. The bill also depended on an administrative arrangement even more complicated than that found in the disability insurance program.

Expanding on the precedent of assigning administrative tasks to bureaucracies outside of the Social Security Administration, the Medicare bill allowed hospitals to transact Medicare business through private intermediaries. Blue Cross served as the model. HEW officials told Mills that "Blue Cross would handle all dealings with hospitals," that the Social Security Administration needed only to do some "spotchecking," rather than extensive auditing.

Like community Blue Cross plans, Medicare reimbursed the hospitals according to their "reasonable costs." Although apparently innocuous, the decision to follow this reimbursement pattern granted considerable power to the hospitals because it meant that hospitals would determine how much it cost to serve the elderly and the federal government would come up with the cash. As a consequence, the federal government, acting like a private employer, purchased medical care rather than trying to control it. The government ran a group plan for the elderly; the employers' plans covered people of working ages.

The American Hospital Association and others who watched out for the hospitals' interests made sure that the Medicare bill protected hospitals. Congress went out of its way to define "reasonable costs" in a way that guaranteed that competent hospitals would not lose money on Medicare. Hospitals should not be deterred, in the words of the Senate Committee on Finance, "from trying to provide the best of modern care," and should be allowed to recover both direct and indirect costs, including depreciation of buildings and equipment, the costs of capital indebtedness, and a portion of the net costs of educational activities, such as stipends for teachers.

Even with these concessions, the Social Security Administration faced formidable opposition from the doctors. It took an external push, the tragic death of John F. Kennedy in 1963, and good political fortune, the election of a heavily Democratic Congress in 1964, to put Medicare over the top. At the end of 1964, Wilbur Mills finally conceded Medicare's inevitability.

Although the American Medical Association continued to argue for a welfare program, the Republicans produced the most serious counterproposal to Medicare. Put forward by Representative John Byrnes of Wisconsin, the plan relied on a combination of general revenues and direct contributions from the elderly, with no one being forced to participate. Those who signed up received a much wider range of services than the Democrats promised in Medicare. Where Medicare was limited to hospital care, the Byrnes plan also included doctors' bills.

Mills then proceeded to astound policy observers when, early in 1965, he recommended adoption of each of the plans. First, he decided to broaden the Kerr-Mills program and create Medicaid. Second, he agreed to support the Byrnes proposal for the coverage of doctors' bills. Third, he acquiesced to the Medicare bill.

The completed bill, one of the most complicated ever contemplated, included the three components of health insurance, and features related to welfare, old-age insurance, and disability insurance. Passed thirty years after the original Social Security Act, it duplicated the 1935 bill's broad scope and cautious approach.

Just as the 1935 Social Security Act relied heavily on public assistance, rather than social insurance, to cope with immediate social problems, so the 1965 Medicare law extended the public assistance system. Medicaid involved new federal grants to the states for health insurance. The states in turn could use the money to start health programs for dependent children, the elderly, the blind, and the "permanently and totally disabled" on welfare or poor enough to qualify as "medically indigent." The new program, therefore, extended the old Kerr-Mills program. Where Kerr-Mills restricted its benefits to the elderly, Medicaid covered other groups among the "deserving poor," the groups who already benefited from welfare programs authorized in the Social Security Act.

Medicaid met with little opposition because both the conservative AMA and the liberal Social Security Administration favored it. For the American Medical Association, Medicaid owed its legitimacy to its close resemblance to Eldercare, the AMA's own proposal for health insurance. Indeed, the association had long favored working with the local authorities who ran welfare programs and who restricted benefits to poor people who would otherwise be unable to pay the doctor.

The Social Security Administration and the newly created Welfare Administration recognized that dependent children and their pregnant mothers needed medical assistance every bit as much as the elderly did. Hence, they had been working on a program similar to Medicaid for a number of years. Their only reservations centered on the relationship between Medicaid and Medicare: they wanted to be sure that the passage of Medicaid did not foreclose the adoption of Medicare. Mills's bill reassured them on this point and gained their favor.

The second element of the Mills plan involved the acceptance of the Byrnes proposal to cover doctors' bills. Since the Byrnes proposal had originated as antagonistic, rather than complementary to Medicare, this element of the package occasioned the greatest surprise. As proposed, it covered hospital and doctors' bills; as modified by Mills, it was limited to doctors' bills.

The forced marriage of the Byrnes bill, which some had dubbed "bettercare," and Medicare satisfied Mills and gained the quick acceptance of Wilbur Cohen and the Johnson administration as well. The advantage to Mills consisted of taking some of the burden of health care costs off the shoulders of the Social Security system. Social Security would have to meet the costs of hospital care, but doctors' bills could be paid from other sources of revenue, such as general revenues and contributions from the beneficiaries themselves. And to appease the doctors, coverage for doctors' bills could be voluntary rather than compulsory. Liberals in the health insurance coalition, for whom the method of administering health insurance was never as important as the range of benefits offered, delighted in the fact that the legislation now covered doctors' bills. During discussion of previous versions of Medicare, Connecticut senator Abraham Ribicoff had warned President Johnson that Medicare would "disillusion millions of the nation's elderly. Too many believe *all* of their medical bills will be paid, not just the hospital and related charges." Mills remedied that.

Wilbur Cohen was not terribly surprised by Mills's legislative sleight-of-hand, and some Washington insiders, who had watched Cohen over the years, secretly believed that Cohen himself had suggested the blending of "bettercare" and Medicare. Whether that was true or not, Cohen, on behalf of the administration, accepted the compromise with alacrity. As a highly placed assistant to Cohen later explained, "no one thought that Medicare would be permanent. We regarded it as a temporary arrangement." When things got rearranged, Medicare "Part B," as the Byrnes proposal came to be known, might be folded into the Social Security program. As matters stood, elderly people paid for it through reductions in their Social Security checks. It seemed a small matter to change that detail and have working people prepay their doctors' bills through deductions in their paychecks.

Part B of Medicare looked anomalous, as though it were a complete break with the past, a new way of doing social policy. Yet, as Wilbur Cohen realized, an analogue between the Byrnes proposal and the original Social Security Act existed. Just as the 1935 Social Security bill contained a proposal for "voluntary" annuities, so the 1965 bill featured a voluntary health insurance program. In 1935, the life insurance companies and the general indifference toward social insurance defeated the voluntary annuity proposal; in 1965, the voluntary health insurance proposal gained the active support of the Republicans and the passive support of the Democrats. It passed.

The third and final part of the Mills master compromise on health insurance involved his acceptance of Medicare. Mills accepted Medicare in part because of political pressure and in part because he now thought that hospital insurance was hedged with enough protections to make it viable. Congress accepted the Mills legislation gratefully and made only a few changes. Lyndon Johnson signed the bill in an emotional ceremony that took place in Independence, Missouri, home of a still vigorous Harry Truman. At the ceremony, two living politicians saluted two dead ones. The object of John F. Kennedy's 1960 pilgrimage to FDR's grave had finally been realized.

After twenty-five years of active campaigning by Social Security advocates, the program now included hospital insurance. Just as the 1935 Social Security Act, the original source of social welfare legislation, began old-age insurance, so the Medicare legislation, the second source of social welfare legislation, initiated hospital insurance.

Much had changed, however, since the era when the senior John Dingell was a member of Congress. The Medicare legislation had not so much the bold qualities of the 1943 Wagner-Murray-Dingell bill as the tentative quality of the original Social Security proposals. Indeed, the new legislation fit neatly into the health care consensus. Through its benefits formula, it focused on hospitals, rather than on other treatment centers. Through its reimbursement features, it contributed federal support for hospital construction, medical research, and medical education. Through the use of Blue Cross and other fiscal intermediaries, the law reinforced the local nature of health care finance. It was, in short, a passive form of intervention into the market for medical care, a fringe benefit for the elderly.

The postwar social welfare consensus reached its high-water mark in 1965. Passage of Medicare signaled a cease fire between the government and the forces of private medical care, whose ranks included the American Medical Association, the insurance companies, community Blue Cross plans, and the hospitals. Under the terms of the cease fire, the government agreed to provide for the medical needs of the elderly and the poor, and the private medical care financiers and providers continued to serve the rest of the population. Already, however, events were under way that would put considerable strain on the system.

The Complexities of Health Insurance

On closer examination, the line separating the public and private sectors of the health care industry proved to be illusory. The federal government, ostensibly in charge of Medicare and Medicaid, ceded many of its administrative responsibilities to the states, who ran Medicaid programs for the poor, and many of its financial responsibilities to Blue Cross and Blue Shield plans, who played an important role in the management of Medicare. The government itself provided no actual care. Instead, it left responsibility for providing care to local hospitals and doctors. At the same time, the private system depended on construction funds, research funds, and other subsidies from the government, as well as on tax laws that were favorable to employers who financed the health care of their employees. Health care, in short, was a very complicated industry, with national, local, private, and public components.

Despite this complexity, many advocates of national health insurance, refreshed by the passage of Medicare, kept their eyes on the ultimate prize of national health insurance. Medicare made the mechanics of national health insurance easier to envision: start by collecting money for Medicare and then increase the payroll contributions by some small fraction and begin a national health insurance program for people of all ages. National health insurance, for the first time, came to be viewed as an incremental expansion of Social Security, rather than as something that lay beyond a threshold that politicians feared to cross. Congress had, after all, crossed the threshold with Medicare. It was now a matter of a few more steps.

After 1965, the complexity of the health care industry conflicted with the simplicity of the national health insurance vision. Eventually this conflict led to the demise of comprehensive national health insurance and exposed another aspect of the welfare state crisis. What is apparent in retrospect was, however, far from clear in the years between 1965 and 1972. The growth of social welfare programs in general and of medical programs in particular characterized social policy in those years.

Steady incremental expansion in health care policy culminated in major new legislation in 1972, when Congress amended the Social Security Act to provide an entitlement to Medicare for disabled individuals. In addition, Congress created a special entitlement to medical care for people with kidney disease who required kidney dialysis.

In the era of comprehensive reform proposals, in the manner of President Nixon's Family Assistance Plan, national health insurance advocates did not lack for grand schemes. In 1969 and 1970, Senator Edward Kennedy, who regarded health care as his area of special expertise and as an appropriate way to maintain the social concerns of his brothers John and Robert, put forward a plan that would have provided free health care to most individuals. So serious was the possibility of the passage of national health insurance that President Nixon felt obligated to counter with a plan of his own. Nixon's plan, which relied on a strategy that came to be called "mandating," required employers to provide a minimum package of health insurance benefits to their employees.

Just as in welfare reform, however, the issue in health insurance was already shifting from insuring access to controlling the costs of care. And that inevitably brought policymakers face-to-face with the realities of the health care industry and the near impossibility of effectively regulating it.

In the first place, regulation was the exact thing that the AMA had feared before Medicare's passage. If the government were to begin setting prices for the doctors' services, the doctors' worst fears would have come true. Hence, the doctors protected their professional autonomy from government intrusion, limiting the effectiveness of any regulatory effort.

In the second place, regulation was an economic term being applied to a field that many considered to be beyond the reach of economic theory. If one believed that a human life was priceless, then it became hard to envision the rationing of medical care. Many of the decisions in health care, in other words, carried moral and ethical overtones that made the imposition of regulatory controls difficult.

In the third place, the very complexity of the health care industry defeated regulatory efforts. Insurance companies, for example, continued to be regulated at the state rather than the federal level. In 1945, Congress reasserted the right of states, rather than the federal government, to regulate the insurance industry, and the insurance companies fought hard to preserve state control over regulation. Blue Cross plans also depended on state, rather than federal, legislative authority. It would be extremely difficult for the federal government to cut across the conflicting lines of authority and regulate the health care industry, even if it could identify this industry with precision. For example, did one want to regulate providers or financiers, hospitals or doctors?

Although the federal government lacked an easy means to regulate the costs of medical care, it soon found itself playing an important role in health care finance. Further, rising medical costs became defined as federal problems, until, at some point, the control of costs became as important as the passage of national health insurance.

Health insurance became expensive very quickly. In old-age insurance, a gradual building up of costs unfolded over many years. Although Social Security planners spoke of reserve funds that would grow to more than $40 billion in 1980, they dealt with much smaller levels of funds, on the order of half a billion dollars, when the program began operations in 1937. Medicare and Medicaid had no grace period before they faced large expenditures, since people received care almost as soon as the program went into effect. The total cost of that care reflected the cost of medical care, as much as the number of elderly or poor people in the population. The government simply agreed, particularly in the Medicare program, to pay prevailing rates to doctors and actual costs to the hospitals.

Thus, even in the era of program expansion, Congress began to complain about the costs of the medical programs, and the grumbling grew with the passing years. As early as 1967, Congress passed legislation designed to limit Medicaid expenditures, and it followed this law with provisions in 1972 that allowed the states to institute programs in which the Medicaid patients themselves paid part of the costs of their care. In that year as well, Congress created Professional Standards Review Organizations, intended to monitor the quality and utilization of services, in the hope of reducing the costs of care by cutting down on unnecessary medical procedures.

Costs just continued to rise. Medical care costs, although rising in the seven years before Medicare was passed, rose twice as fast in the first five years after its passage. Meanwhile, the federal government became the largest single payer of medical care in the country.

The statistics could make a person dizzy. In 1965, the nation spent about 6.2 percent of its gross national product on health care; 75 percent of those expenditures were private and the remainder public (local, state, and federal). In 1970, the percentage of GNP devoted to health care rose to 7.6, despite a substantial rise in the level of GNP itself. Meanwhile, the private share fell to 63.5 percent. By 1983, health care costs consumed nearly 11 percent of the GNP, with public expenditures accounting for 42 percent of those costs. Looked at more broadly, the federal share in the payment of health care costs grew from 13 to 29 percent between 1950 and 1985, and between 1966 and 1980 the costs of Medicare and Medicaid doubled every four years.

Almost all of the interested parties paid an increasing amount for medical care. In 1984, for example, employer contributions amounted to $1,549 per insured employee, an expense that equalled 7.4 percent of the payroll. Private health insurance premiums reached $100 billion in 1983, more than three-quarters of which were paid by employers. Meanwhile, outlays for Medicare totaled about $70 billion in fiscal year 1987 (compared with $7.1 billion in 1970), and outlays for Medicaid reached $26 billion in fiscal 1987 (compared with $2.7 billion in 1970).

These statistics trace the results of what historian Bernard Bailyn has called "latent" events that unfolded over a period of time and played an important role in policy outcomes but were not specific events that reflected a discrete occurrence. No one law or single event led to the rise in medical care costs; instead a seemingly infinite number of small events, occurring within a system that was beyond any single person's comprehension or control, produced the rise.

The rise in costs nonetheless exercised a pervasive influence over the national health insurance debate. By the end of the 1970s, for example, nearly all health insurance proposals attempted to contain health care costs, forcing them to reconcile the goals of making more people eligible for health insurance and keeping costs within reasonable limits. When Edward Kennedy put forward a new health insurance proposal in 1978, for example, the scheme allowed private health plans to compete for subscribers, in the hope of promoting efficiency and lowering costs. In an effort to set an upper limit on the nation's health budget, Kennedy also proposed fixed rates for care and other budget constraints.

Despite this effort, the senator failed to "thread the needle," to use Kennedy's phrase, of national health insurance. By the late 1970s, the health care debate, like the welfare reform debate, was going on in an atmosphere of perceived failure. The government spent more and more money on health care and still many people lacked health insurance. Existing programs, once perceived to be major accomplishments that broke the impasse over health policy, were now widely regarded as flawed, as obstacles to the attainment of comprehensive reform.

In health care, as in welfare reform, something happened to the nature of reform. What began as a moral issue in the 1930s eventually became a technical issue in the 1970s. The health care system reached a point where, even more than the welfare system, it could not be comprehended without reference to statistics. As economist Rashi Fein puts it, "For those who designed possible programs and debated how to implement them, or even whether they could be implemented, the national health insurance debate called for equations, not emotions, for symposia, not sermons." National health insurance reports, like welfare reform proposals, began to read like "engineering manuals." It became much more difficult to rally people to the cause of national health insurance. In the end, the effort, like that of comprehensive welfare reform, was quietly abandoned.

Incremental Cost Containment

As with welfare reform, comprehensive health policy reform eventually gave way to incremental reform in the programs over which the federal government had the most control; and, nearly always, the incremental reforms featured devices to control costs. Similarly, each player in the health policy debate worked with the small piece of the health care system that was under his control. As a result, employers and state governments each played a role in incremental reform.

Employers, for their part, banded together to learn ways of reducing their health care costs, such as by increasing the employees' share of the costs. For example, in 1980 only 5 percent of employer health care plans required a deductible greater than $100; in 1985, 43 percent did so. Meanwhile, the employees also paid more of the basic cost of health insurance. In the late 1980s, the Service Employees International Union discovered that the employees' contributions for health insurance were increasing twice as fast as the employers' contributions.

Devices such as wellness campaigns, employers encouraging healthy practices such as stopping smoking and limiting alcohol consumption, also became popular. Companies discovered that they could save even more money by monitoring their own health care claims rather than turning health insurance over to a private company. In the jargon of the field, many companies engaged in "utilization review," making sure that employees received only appropriate services and that employees went to only cost-efficient (cheaper) providers to receive the services. All of these practices amounted to what the health insurance trade association called a revolution in "managed care."

The managed care revolution extended to the choices of health care providers available to employers and employees. Instead of an open-ended arrangement between providers and consumers, in which the providers kept a running tab, the new arrangements, which took such specific forms as "health maintenance organizations" (HMOs) and "preferred provider arrangements," involved fixed fees. An organization agreed to provide a wide range of services for a fixed sum of money. If an employee was well or was afraid to go the doctor, the organization made money. If the person was frequently seeing doctors or in the hospital, the organization lost money.

Not all consumers embraced this form of medicine. By 1987 only about one out of every six insured individuals received care in the new types of plans. Some employees complained that the plans restricted individual choice, because people did not have the privilege of choosing their physician. Instead, they were required to go to a doctor who agreed to accept reimbursement from the plan or, in a strictly managed health maintenance organization, to a doctor who worked for the HMO. Often the plan did not allow them to see a doctor at all, preferring that they confer, preferably by telephone, with a nurse-practitioner, who, by seeing less severe cases, saved the doctor's time and the plan's expense. Much of the cost savings achieved by these organizations depended on restricting hospital admissions. That, in turn, led to disagreements between patient and physician over the severity of a particular illness.

Prepaid group practice, in other words, involved a degree of rationing in the amount of service a person received and in the time the person spent with a doctor. As such, it reflected a new, cost-conscious form of medicine that came to interest employers and others who paid the bills.

States, for their part, also tried to deal with the piece of the health system over which they had some control. Maryland, for example, passed legislation in 1971 that allowed the state to set hospital rates. Slowly, the state worked out the regulatory problems. First came a review of the rates being charged by Maryland's hospitals. Then the state applied to the Medicare program for a special "waiver" from existing Medicare rules. Federal authorities granted the waiver on one important condition: that the state agree to keep the percentage increase in cost per hospital admission below the national average.

Beginning on January 1, 1977, Maryland initiated its "all payer" system. Three issues dominated the rate-setting process. One was the special discount received by Blue Cross. Blue Cross, for reasons related to politics and history, paid only about 90 percent of what commercial health insurance companies paid for the same care. Blue Cross wanted to retain its special advantage over its competitors, and commercial insurers hoped to use the rate-setting process as a way of ending the Blue Cross discount.

A second issue was the growing cost generated by people who went into the hospital without health insurance. Increasingly, such cases became dead-weight losses, "bad debts" or charity cases. The hospitals wanted some way to allocate these costs to third-party payers with cash at their disposal.

The third issue was the rising cost of health care itself. To keep the plan in existence, the state had to limit increases in health care costs and keep them below the national average.

State authorities tried to deal with the competing interests of organizations that financed health care, the growing need to subsidize health care for the poor, and the policy goal of slowing down the rate of increase in hospital costs. The Maryland Health Services Cost Review Commission eventually endorsed a system that allowed each hospital to recover some of its bad debts and that narrowed, but did not eliminate, the difference between what Blue Cross paid and what commercial insurers paid. Beyond these accommodations to the politics of health care finance, the commission tried to replace a system based strictly on costs—what a hospital actually spent—with a system based on reasonable costs—what the commission deemed reasonable for a hospital to have spent. The state, in other words, tried to distinguish between an open-ended system and a system that set some limits on the amount a hospital would pay for each admission.

New York faced even more acute problems than did Maryland. For example, by 1975, New York City stood on the brink of financial disaster, and that put pressure on the Medicaid program. New York City, which helped to finance and administer the state's Medicaid program, lacked the money to keep Medicaid income eligibility levels current with the rate of inflation. That meant fewer poor people qualified for Medicaid. When these people became hospital patients— and many of them were in hospitals run by the city itself—they became bad debts. Hospitals responded by raising their charges to commercial health insurance companies. Even so, hospitals with high Medicaid caseloads, such as New York's municipal hospitals, continued to face severe problems, since they had relatively few commercial payers on which to unload their bad debts. Meanwhile, private insurers objected to being singled out for higher rates, as their rates became double those paid by Medicare, Medicaid, and Blue Cross, each of which benefited from legal protections that kept their rates at relatively low levels. In retaliation, some commercial insurers refused to sell new health insurance policies in New York. The entire health care financing system threatened to unravel.

New York followed Maryland's lead and established an all payer system, beginning in 1982. The New York approach also mandated special surcharges, to finance what became known as "uncompensated care." In addition, these funds provided special relief to financially distressed hospitals, such as the municipal hospitals in New York City.

Massachusetts took the state approach to incremental reform to

The Mirage of National Health Insurance

its limits in 1988. Governor Michael Dukakis, in the middle of a successful effort to achieve the Democratic presidential nomination, signed a new health law in April. A complicated piece of legislation, in the manner of the other state laws, it called for the eventual achievement of universal access to health care for the citizens of Massachusetts through such measures as mandating coverage for the employed and providing new coverage for the poor. Almost as soon as the law went into effect, however, fiscal problems appeared that put the eventual achievement of the law's goals into doubt.

Nonetheless, the Massachusetts law represented an important milestone in the history of health insurance policy. It appeared, for the first time since the late 1930s, that the states, rather than the federal government, were taking the lead in this area, just as they were on welfare reform. States with relatively strong economies, such as Massachusetts and New Jersey, attempted to use their newly rediscovered wealth to resolve the enduring problems of controlling health care costs and providing access to care. The states, true to their heritage in the insurance field, took what observers called a "regulatory" approach to the problem.

Meanwhile, the federal government, having lost the initiative in health insurance, still needed to attend to the problems in the Medicare program. National health insurance, like comprehensive welfare reform, had received its last hurrah from the Carter administration. Members of the Reagan administration, who wanted to clear national health insurance from the national agenda, felt no qualms about abandoning it.

The Reagan administration eventually endorsed and Congress accepted an important change in Medicare. This change, legislated as part of the comprehensive Social Security bill in 1983, marked an attempt to put an effective limit on hospital costs. Something known as a "diagnosis related group" (DRG) served as the chosen device. Assume, for example, that a hospital performed a hysterectomy. Under the old system, the hospital kept a running tab on its costs—bandages, nursing care, syringes, medicines—and then billed the local Medicare representative (who, more often than not, worked for Blue Cross). In theory at least, the higher the tab, the more money returned to the hospital. It was like putting a hotel bill on someone else's credit card and making long distance calls and ordering room service, secure in the knowledge that you would not have to pay. Under the new system, a hysterectomy fell into a particular diagnosis related group, and the hospital received a predetermined amount for it. The efficient hospital, the one that whisked a woman quickly out the door, stood to make more money than the less efficient hospital that allowed the woman to run up a large bill. The DRG system, unlike the old free-spending plan, resembled receiving a per diem and being told to pick your own hotel.

The Reagan administration, then, endorsed a regulatory strategy that resembled what the states, such as Maryland, that used Medicare waivers had been doing. It opted for prospective reimbursement rather than cost-based, retrospective reimbursement. Although the change applied only to hospital costs and not to doctors' bills and although some hospitals, such as rehabilitation facilities and mental hospitals, were not covered, the law set an important precedent. It was as though the federal government had finally discovered its power in the medical market. As the largest single payer, the government carried regulatory clout, and implementation of the diagnosis related group system showed that the Reagan administration was not afraid of using it.

This, of course, was the sort of thing that the hospitals and doctors had feared all along. Once let into the medical market, the federal government would insist on regulating it. Ironically, Ronald Reagan and the Republicans, rather than Wilbur Cohen and the Democrats, were the ones who implemented the change. Something like the political dynamic that enabled Richard Nixon, arch anticommunist, to go to China applied here as well. The Republicans could make regulatory overtures denied to the Democrats.

Even though employers cut down on medical costs, states took innovative steps to regulate hospital charges, and the federal government regulated the Medicare program, a fundamental problem remained. Some people still lacked health insurance, and received either no care or care paid for by others.

The problem of the uninsured became particularly acute during the Reagan recovery in the mid-1980s. As more people became employed, more people also became uninsured. That incongruity implied a fundamental failure of the public policy understanding that private employers financed health care for the working population. If employment were no longer synonymous with what might be called health security, that meant an important part of America's welfare state was coming unglued. The figures indicated that 35 million Americans were without health insurance in 1985. Thirty-two percent of the uninsured worked full time; 30 percent lived in families headed by full-time workers, and 11 percent of the uninsured held part-time jobs that lasted from 18 to 34 hours a week. The retail trades and service industries employed nearly half of the working uninsured, and the majority of the working uninsured labored in firms with fewer than 100 employees. Only two-thirds of the firms with fewer than 100 employees offered health insurance.

Many of the uninsured, as many as 32 percent, earned incomes that fell below the poverty line; and over half of those people, or 19 percent of all the uninsured, belonged to one of the groups eligible for Medicaid. Although their incomes put them below the poverty line, they still made too much money to qualify for Medicaid in their particular state. As a result, neither the government nor private employers subsidized health care for such people, a major gap in America's safety net and a major shortcoming of America's welfare state.

When Reagan left office, the problem of the uninsured rivaled the problem of health care cost containment as a difficult one on the policy agenda. Policymakers, mindful of the need to work out solutions that respected the complexity of the health care market, proposed various combinations of mandated coverages aimed at employers who did not offer health insurance, combined with expansions of the Medicaid program for the poor and the near poor.

Health Care and the Crisis of the Welfare State

Health care fit the general pattern that applied to Social Security and welfare. Using the framework of the Social Security Act, the nation had by 1965 arrived at what was regarded as a permanent solution to financing health care. Although some people wanted to change the terms of this solution to provide national health insurance for people of all ages, they soon found their proposals overwhelmed by the perceived failure to control the growth of the existing programs. Just as the cost of maintaining the Social Security and welfare programs came to be perceived as prohibitive, so the size of the cost blocked the expansion of the welfare state to cover national health insurance.

The crisis arose from the fact that, just as no one could figure out how to take welfare recipients off the rolls, so health care cost containment looked impossible to achieve. The nation's apparent failure to regulate the health care industry meant that some people could not afford health care, and that implied, at the very least, that their health care was being seriously neglected. Babies who lacked prenatal and pediatric health care because their parents failed to qualify for health insurance suffered particularly severe consequences.

Still, even as the welfare reform debate reached some sort of a climax in 1988, the health insurance problem retained its status as the Mount Everest of social reform. The difference between 1970 and

1988 was that the problem no longer had the quality of an invigorating challenge; it now seemed a task that was just too daunting. Consensus, in this most scientific and technologically driven of fields, had yielded to crisis, just as it had in the nation's social insurance and welfare programs.

★ ★ ★
_____
IV

Conclusion

Long-Term Care of the Welfare State

Failed expectations, matched by a paralysis of government institutions, produced the crisis of the welfare state. "The hope behind this
statute," Justice Benjamin Cardozo wrote in 1937, referring to the
Social Security Act, "is to save men and women from the rigors of
the poorhouse as well as from the haunting fear that such a lot awaits
them when journey's end is near." In America, despite the self-confidence generated by the mid-twentieth century consensus in social
welfare policy, the haunting fear remains a pressing reality in the
1990s.

Until Tobe Trickle reached 86 and developed Alzheimer's disease,
he did fine. Then Edrell Trickle put him in a nursing home. First,
she placed him in a nice facility near their home in Arkansas, but
soon the relentlessly arriving bills, which very quickly amounted to
over $60,000, forced her to move him to a cheaper place in Missouri.
Like nearly everyone else, the Trickles faced the nursing home bills
without the help of Medicare or private insurance. Tobe Trickle lost
first his mind and then his life in a poorhouse; he and his wife knew
Cardozo's haunting fear.

In the summer of 1988, a national effort to pass long-term care
legislation emerged. Groups such as the American Association of
Retired Persons, the Villers Foundation, and the Save Our Security
Coalition—all of whom belonged to a loosely defined lobby that
pushed for laws in aid of the elderly—joined together to create "Long-
Term Care '88." The group proclaimed long-term care an "idea that
can elect the next President." Throughout the election year, the group
attempted to highlight the issue, pressuring each of the presidential

candidates to declare his approval of new legislation to ease the financial burden of paying for long-term care.

By the summer of 1988, long-term care shaped up as one of the Capitol's major political fights. A piece of legislation known as the Pepper bill, after its main sponsor Claude Pepper, the 87-year-old former senator and now chairman of the House Rules Committee, served as the specific vehicle. Described by the *Washington Post* as a "revered champion of the elderly," Pepper wanted to extend health insurance for the elderly to include new home health and personal care benefits, and, as Jim Slattery, a Democrat from Kansas, put it, "Who wants to be out there voting against Claude Pepper in an election year?"

Although Pepper's bill would cost perhaps $14 billion a year, he planned to finance it in a time-honored manner by raising the Social Security taxes of Americans making more than $45,000 a year. The bill served both as a tribute to Senator Pepper and as a means of reinforcing a long American tradition of using the Social Security system to solve social problems.

This tradition now spanned half a century, beginning in 1935 with the passage of the Social Security Act and the initiation of unemployment compensation and old-age insurance programs, which were the first large-scale efforts to make unemployment and retirement public responsibilities. Both workers and employers set aside money that was then used to pay benefits to laid-off or retired workers.

The old-age insurance part of the program became an unexpected success because it proved remarkably adaptable to the conditions of the postwar world. The creators of the Social Security Act were working in a political, if not an intellectual, vacuum when they resisted pressures to create programs of immediate advantage to the unemployed. Distrustful of programs under the active management of Congress, the creators recommended a social insurance approach instead. Congress, wishing to do something in aid of the elderly and unemployed and not wanting to oppose the administration, reluctantly went along with these suggestions and passed old-age insurance and unemployment compensation, in addition to the more popular welfare programs.

With the exception of President Roosevelt and Labor Secretary Perkins, no initial demand for social security on the part of influential policymakers preceded the legislation; instead reformers, motivated by a strong belief in social insurance and professionalism, used the financial emergency created by the Depression to advance a progressive agenda of longstanding duration. Deliberations over Social

Security became a forum in which to reenact old arguments over the fine points of social insurance. Should, for example, there be employers' reserves in unemployment compensation or pooled funds? Not much interested in social insurance to begin with, policymakers showed even less desire to debate its fine points. They made snap decisions on the basis of political expediency, as when they turned the details of unemployment compensation over to the states.

After 1935, legislators continued to ignore Social Security. If it entered the realm of public discourse at all, it served as a conventional partisan issue. Republicans ridiculed the elaborate procedures for protecting its financial integrity; Democrats responded with comments about the Republicans' lack of social concern. Interest in state welfare programs and in the Townsend plan remained high. Nothing guaranteed Social Security's survival during those years, and another program could easily have replaced it.

Social Security's survival can, in retrospect, be traced to legislative inertia and bureaucratic self-interest. Congress hesitated to put any program out of business, because to do so inevitably incurred someone's displeasure. It proved easier, then, to work around old-age insurance and to concentrate on increasing welfare payments to the elderly. Furthermore, the employees of the Social Security Board firmly regarded social insurance as superior to welfare and took what steps they could to insure its survival. The 1939 amendments proved crucial in this regard: a neat accommodation of bureaucratic and political interests that resulted in lower Social Security taxes, higher benefits, and new forms of family benefits.

The war also acted as a brake on the creation of new federal programs and, as such, served to protect the old-age insurance program. During the war years, policymakers, distracted by practical questions related to war management and mobilization, lacked the time or interest to mount a major new social welfare initiative. The war, in effect, preserved certain federal social welfare programs, such as Social Security, even as it ended public works programs such as the WPA, and signaled a major change in the economy that pointed the way to the optimism of the postwar era.

In the changed conditions of the postwar era, the expansion of welfare programs and the enactment of the Townsend Plan faded as social welfare goals. Interest in old-age insurance revived, particularly after the technical terms of expansion were worked out in the 1950 amendments and after major industries, such as the automobile industry, began to implement large-scale pension plans. Also, a resurgence of interest in the rehabilitation approach to social policy occurred, as indicated by local efforts to end juvenile delinquency and hire the handicapped and by major expansions of social services in welfare programs.

The progressive agenda of the Social Security Act, once out of step with current events, acquired a new relevance. Methods of planned savings for the future as embodied in social insurance programs once again meshed with the temper of the times. Methods of psychological adjustment, fashionable in the 1920s, became fashionable once again. Improved economic conditions bred a self-confidence that led directly to the mid-century consensus on social welfare policy.

Between 1941 and 1972, the growing economy created an optimistic sense that the nations' social welfare programs could be solved by social insurance for the working population and rehabilitation for nearly everyone else. Economic growth in and of itself heightened the possibilities of reaching new social goals, such as the participation of women and blacks in the economic mainstream. Indeed, many of the policy efforts of the postwar era focused on facilitating this participation. Some of the efforts took the form of civil rights laws aimed at the prejudices that limited the wages of women and members of minority groups. Others took the form of rehabilitation: advice, training, medical services, all designed to remove the physical and psychological barriers that limited a person's labor force participation.

The mid-century consensus relied on a grand design that made social insurance the major form of American social policy. Social insurance depended on an orderly partnership between private employers and the federal government. Employers handled the costs of health care, and private employers and the federal government, working together, financed the costs of retirement. The grand design reduced social policy to three major objectives: the encouragement of employment, through macroeconomic policy; the maintenance and expansion of Social Security, through competent administration and passage of disability insurance and Medicare; and the rehabilitation of those outside of the labor force, through professionally applied social services.

To be sure, other concerns intruded and momentarily disturbed the consensus. Americans, engaged in a race with the Russians to win the Cold War, worried about the inadequacy of their school systems, about an economic system producing tail fins on cars at the expense of socially valuable products, and about the deterioration of the largest American cities. Nonetheless, the prevailing view in the 1950s and early 1960s cast these and other problems in the form of agreeable challenges for which the nation would soon find solutions.

Little about the various problems challenged the terms of the grand design.

Events between 1950 and 1965 only confirmed the wisdom of the grand design. Economists learned how to fine-tune the economy so as to reduce the rate of recession. Social workers benefited from major new legislative initiatives, such as the Public Welfare Amendments of 1962 and the Economic Opportunity Act of 1964, that gave them the necessary funding and professional training to tackle the problems of those on the edges of the labor market. Lyndon Johnson broke the legislative deadlock and forced Congress to pass major new civil rights legislation that furthered the integration of blacks through the orderly process of law. Women joined the labor force in record numbers after 1964 and participated in a quiet social revolution. After a concerted campaign, Congress extended the Social Security program so that it paid money to disabled people who needed to retire before age 65 and so that it helped to pay the medical bills of the elderly and the disabled. This campaign resulted in the passage of disability insurance in 1956 and of Medicare in 1965.

During the era of the mid-century consensus, old-age insurance proved so successful that the people who ran the program started to think of using the program to promote new social goals. Program administrators and their allies turned their attention to increasing the level of benefits, and in 1972 Congress agreed to raise benefits so that they would keep pace with the rising cost of living. That left Social Security advocates free to explore new ways of using the system, new ways of spending the money deducted from workers' wages.

Following a seductive logic, social insurance advocates chose long-term care as the next step. It formed part of a neat and orderly progression the went from old age and unemployment, to disability, to health care, and finally to long-term care, or disability in old-age. "In the next ten to twenty years," said Wilbur Cohen in 1986, "the crisis in long-term care will reach a crescendo, and in the next cycle of reform something will be done to remedy the situation." The Pepper bill responded to the perception of urgency in the need for a remedy.

Even as Cohen spoke, the mid-century consensus no longer applied, and the grand design no longer governed American social policy. In part, the change reflected changing economic conditions. In the 1970s, the expected trade-off between inflation and unemployment failed to materialize, and a condition known as stagflation, characterized by rising prices and growing unemployment, developed. The economy failed to expand at its previous pace, and families no longer experienced rising standards of living as a matter of course.

In constant (1983) dollars, a married couple earned a "median" money income of $26,982 in 1970 and $26,856 in 1982. Between 1973 and 1974 and again between 1974 and 1975, the gross national product failed to grow enough to counter the inflation rate, and "real" GNP declined.

Since the grand design depended so heavily on economic growth, the absence of this growth created a sense of crisis. Expectations generated by the initial successes of Social Security, the American system of financing health care, and even the welfare system failed to be met. Instead, the economic downturn of the 1970s and early 1980s produced a sense of pessimism. The economy no longer appeared resilient enough to sustain a growing labor force and to accommodate the demands of blacks and women for jobs, dooming a social welfare system that depended on people working and participating in the social insurance programs. Rising prices insidiously undermined the adequacy of social welfare benefits and, combined with persistent unemployment, made the achievement of rehabilitation-related goals difficult.

Even for those people working regularly, the system began to break down. Because Social Security came to depend on current economic conditions, it nearly went bankrupt in the stagflation era. Young working people stopped expressing confidence in the Social Security program and no longer appeared convinced that generous benefits would be there for them. This loss of confidence weakened support for Social Security and hence for the keystone of the consensus. The accomplishment of truly difficult social tasks, such as funding the retirement of the baby boom generation, became that much more difficult to achieve in such an atmosphere. People, in doubt about the system's viability, failed to rally behind calls for current restraint and future sacrifice. Social Security's champions pointed to the program's amazing postwar record; Social Security's detractors concentrated on the program's shaky performance during the stagflation era. Consensus no longer came so easily.

The presence of working people without health insurance signaled another major system failure. According to the truce of 1965, employers provided health insurance for the working population and the government financed the health care of the poor and the elderly. But in the 1980s, neither employers nor the government was purchasing health insurance for a significant number of Americans. Because of the rising costs of health insurance, many people simply did not have it. Rising health care costs reflected an inability to control the cost of services and other commodities in the American economy.

The changing tone of expert commentary revealed a lack of agreement about social goals and processes in post-stagflation America. In the 1950s, academic experts had turned their creative energies toward explaining contradictory programs in reassuring ways. In the academic view, Social Security, with its combination of adequacy and equity, represented a creative blend of private initiative and public concern, a perfect example of the triumph of pragmatic social reform over ideological preconceptions. In the 1970s and 1980s, academic experts applied their creative talents to uncovering the contradictions in Social Security and other social welfare programs. In the new academic view, Social Security deceived the public by masking with reassuring public symbols its true nature as a major source of income redistribution, and academics accepted the responsibility of revealing the deception. In the old analysis, academics, who fancied themselves pragmatic realists, engaged in a willing suspension of disbelief. In the new analysis, academics, who saw themselves as committed radical reformers, carefully tested past performances against future claims. Academic experts, despite their claims of objectivity, no more escaped the prevailing optimism of the 1950s and 1960s or the prevailing pessimism of the 1970s and 1980s than did politicians, policymakers, or members of the general public.

As the mid-century consensus broke down and the grand design no longer appeared adequate to solve social problems, the hope that social policy could be conducted in a setting removed from political pressure faded. Uncertainty among experts and policymakers, such as prevailed in the 1930s and again in the 1970s and 1980s, bred disagreements that inevitably led to conflict over the proper course to follow. In the case of Social Security, political pressures became so intense that the details of the 1983 amendments were deliberately worked out in secret, rather than in the public forum of Congress.

The Pepper long-term care bill generated the sort of intense political conflict that had come to characterize social policy discussions in the age of crisis. Ultimately, the bruising battle produced the defeat of the measure, and in its place Congress chose to appoint a commission to investigate the problems of health insurance and long-term care. When Claude Pepper died shortly thereafter, Senator Jay Rockefeller (D-W.Va.) agreed to chair what came to be known as the Pepper Commission, and he soon led the commissioners on a tour of the nation where they met Edrell Trickle, among others. Everyone agreed on the existence of a long-term care problem, but finding a solution proved nearly impossible. The sticking point, with this matter as with so many others, was cost. As David Durenberger, a Minnesota senator and Pepper Commission member, put it, "people simply aren't ready to shoulder the costs of ensuring that every American has access to the health care they need." In the end, although the Pepper Commission agreed on the need for long-term care and health insurance legislation, it left the details of financing the programs vague.

In the case of long-term care, as with the other concerns of the welfare state, the policies of the past no longer commanded automatic acceptance. Social insurance relied on treating social benefits as entitlements, and some conservatives argued that long-term care could not be handled as an entitlement. Long-term care insurance, asserted former Social Security chief actuary Robert J. Myers, "would be like paying unemployment insurance benefits to people who voluntarily left their jobs." In this view, permissive social insurance systems led to rising beneficiary rolls and prohibitive costs.

Myers, for one, believed that, contrary to the grand design, social insurance might not provide the best response to long-term care. Perhaps it made more sense to search for alternatives to institutional care, such as home or community-based remedies and to implement them through some combination of state and private action. This approach, already tried in the 1988 welfare amendments, held the promise of promoting efficiency and saving federal dollars.

Social insurance advocates, for whom such an approach was anathema, believed that previous state and private approaches to social welfare problems had demonstrated only their inefficiency. These advocates pointed to the gaps in the health insurance market and to the obvious fact that any private solution would arrive too late for Tobe Trickle. Social insurance, by way of contrast, solved the problem in a manner that protected the dignity of the individual by not forcing him to undergo a humiliating means test; and, by spreading the considerable costs of long-term care across many people, it lowered individual costs.

The two sides talked past one another; both made sense, and no easy means existed to marry one vision of social policy to the other. In the absence of a resolution of the dispute between the defenders of the grand design and the promoters of a new design, people passed off the costs of social problems where they could. Employers shifted costs to employees; the federal government mandated charges on the states. Small changes in social insurance programs introduced subtle ways of differentiating between the rich and the poor. Disguised forms of a guaranteed income, with deliberately deceptive names like earned income tax credit and food stamps, appeared.

As the experts floundered and the politicians bewailed the situation, no effective substitute for the social insurance and rehabilitation approach emerged. Meanwhile, real problems, such as those

faced by Alzheimer's disease patient Tobe Trickle and welfare grand-
mother Maeola Drakeford, remained to be solved, and real accomplishments, such as the transformation of old age from a time of
economic anxiety to a time of security, threatened to be forgotten.
The nation awaited another era when it could suspend its sense of
disbelief and build a coherent set of social policies on the framework
of consensus.

A Note on the Sources

As academic ventures go, the development of American social welfare programs remains a relatively unexplored topic; so, much of the research for this book inevitably depended on primary sources unavailable to the general reader. These included valuable collections at the big three among social welfare archives: the National Archives (for Social Security and rehabilitation records), the Wisconsin State Historical Society (for the papers of Wilbur Cohen, Edwin Witte, and Arthur Altmeyer), and Social Welfare History Archives at the University of Minnesota (for materials related to the activities of social welfare professionals).

There is, however, an indispensable primary source available to any reader, and that is the material published by the U.S. government. In particular, legislation is almost always accompanied by a very thorough published record, including hearings by the relevant committees, the debate on the floors of the House and Senate, and committee reports that explain the particular legislation, often without resorting to the jargon that obscures much policy discourse. In the case of Social Security, for example, one could go to any government repository and, for any amendment, find hearings conducted by the House Committee on Ways and Means and the Senate Committee on Finance; and one could follow the actual legislative debates by reading the relevant volume of the *Congressional Record*. Most libraries would also include the president's statements related to the bill as part of their collection of presidential documents. Some might have the *Social Security Bulletin*, a monthly magazine published by the Social Security Administration, which routinely reviews legislative developments in Social Security.

General Works

For a general background to the topics discussed in this book, I would recommend three books. For Social Security, one should start and finish with Martha Derthick, *Policymaking for Social Security* (Washington, D.C.: Brookings Institution, 1979), as fine an account of the development of the program as we may ever have. For health insurance and the development of medicine more generally, the key book is Paul Starr, *The Social Transformation of American Medicine* (New York: Basic Books, 1982). Starr manages to synthesize an extraordinary amount of material as he shapes an accessible narrative about the rise of the medical profession in the United States. For welfare, the best book remains Gilbert Y. Steiner, *Social Insecurity: The Politics of Welfare* (Chicago: Rand McNally and Co., 1966). Steiner, like Derthick, is very perceptive about the political environment in which welfare policy has been shaped.

Beyond these essential books, one could assemble a long shelf of excellent books that provide an overview of social welfare policy. One could begin with the topic of poverty and the two durable surveys on the subject. These include James T. Patterson, *America's Struggle Against Poverty 1900–1980* (Cambridge, Mass.: Harvard University Press, 1981) and the earlier Robert Bremner, *From the Depths: The Discovery of Poverty in the United States* (New York: New York University Press, 1956). Donald T. Critchlow and Ellis Hawley have edited a good collection of scholarly articles and primary sources on poverty, *Poverty and Public Policy in Modern America* (Chicago: Dorsey Press, 1989). Within this collection, Carl Brauer's essay on the War on Poverty, reprinted from a scholarly journal, is particularly useful. For the connection between nineteenth-century poorhouses and modern public assistance the best source is Michael Katz, *In the Shadow of the Poorhouse* (New York: Basic Books, 1986). Katz provides more specific data, on such things as how poorhouses operated, in *Poverty and Policy in American History* (New York: Academic Press, 1983) and completes his stunning social welfare trilogy with *The Undeserving Poor: From the War on Poverty to the War on Welfare* (New York: Pantheon Books, 1989), a provocative intellectual history of recent policies. Despite a certain amount of overlap, each of Katz's three volumes can be read with profit. Two overviews of social welfare policy that view change over time from the perspective of social work and social welfare workers, and that are good sources of facts and contain provocative interpretations, are James Leiby, *A History of Social Welfare and Social Work in the United States* (New York: Columbia University Press, 1978) and Walter I. Trattner, *From Poor Law to Welfare State*, 4th ed. (New York: Free Press, 1990). Another interpretive overview of social welfare history and policy that emphasizes the connection between public and private activities, far more than I do in this book, is Edward D. Berkowitz and Kim McQuaid, *Creating the Welfare State: The Political Economy of Twentieth-Century Reform*, 2nd ed. (New York: Praeger Press, 1988).

Each of the major areas of this study—Social Security, health insurance, and welfare—has also generated a small stack of valuable books. On Social Security, W. Andrew Achenbaum has written an excellent history and policy analysis that begins with the creation of the program and ends with practical suggestions for the program's improvement. *Social Security: Visions and Revisions* (New York: Cambridge University Press, 1986) also contains an astonishing set of notes that lists virtually every source on the topic that was then available. One book, written from a Marxist perspective with an appreciation of history and an understanding of sociological theory, unavailable to Achenbaum, is Jill S. Quadagno, *The Transformation of Old Age Security; Class and Politics in the American Welfare State* (Chicago: University of Chicago Press, 1988). Two other useful books examine Social Security from opposing but strangely complementary perspectives. Carolyn L. Weaver, *The Crisis in Social Security* (Durham, N.C.: Duke University Press, 1982) uses public choice theory to show how bureaucrats and others can suppress information and freedom of choice; and Jerry Cates, *Insuring Inequality* (Ann Arbor: University of Michigan Press, 1983) uses more conventional political analysis to show how bureaucrats and others can manipulate public opinion and obscure the emergence of truly radical social programs. William Graebner highlights the Depression-era emphasis on retirement in *A History of Retirement: The Meaning and Function of An American Institution, 1885–1978* (New Haven: Yale University Press, 1980). My contributions to the literature on Social Security include an edited book, *Social Security after Fifty: Successes and Failures* (Westport, Conn.: Greenwood Press, 1987), which contains interpretive essays by Mark Leff, Achenbaum, Derthick, and Henry Aaron, as well as *Disabled Policy: America's Programs for the Handicapped* (New York: Cambridge University Press, 1987), which concentrates on disability insurance. The latter book builds on the political analysis of Deborah Stone, *The Disabled State* (Philadelphia: Temple University Press, 1984).

On health insurance, the best recent interpretation, one that compares the American and the English experiences, is Daniel Fox, *Health Policies, Health Politics* (Princeton: Princeton University Press, 1987). Although health insurance and Medicare have not proved popular topics for historians, many historians have written social histories of particular hospitals and of the hospital itself. The commanding work is Charles E. Rosenberg, *The Care of Strangers: The Rise of America's Hospital System* (New York: Basic Books, 1987), a sensitive portrayal of the hospital's rise to respectability.

Welfare has not produced a similarly long list of solid historical books, in part because it is so controversial. Gilbert Steiner remains the commentator of choice, as in *The State of Welfare* (Washington, D.C.: Brookings Institution, 1971). We await a comprehensive study of modern developments in welfare, in the tradition of Starr on medicine or Derthick on Social Security. Blanche Coll, whose *Perspectives on Public Welfare* (Washington: Government Printing Office, 1969) is an excellent account of nineteenth- and early-twentieth-century developments, is writing such a book, tentatively called "More Than a Salvage Operation." One particularly fine although narrowly focused study is Laurence E. Lynn and David Whitman, *The President as Policymaker: Jimmy Carter and Welfare Reform* (Philadelphia: Temple University Press, 1981).

Preface

For characterizing the intellectual positions of liberals and conservatives, I rely on Daniel Levine, *Poverty and Society: The Growth of the American Welfare State in International Comparison* (New Brunswick, N.J.: Rutgers University Press, 1989), an excellent survey of international developments; on the introduction in Margaret Weir, Ann Shola Orloff, and Theda Skocpol, eds., *The Politics of Social Policy in the United States* (Princeton: Princeton University Press, 1988), a valuable compendium of essays that attempt to "bring the state back into" discussions of social policy; and on Edward J. Harpham and Richard K. Scotch, "Ideology and Welfare Reform in the 1980s," in Richard W. Couglin, ed., *Reforming Welfare: Lessons, Limits, and Choices* (Albuquerque: University of New Mexico Press, 1989).

Chapter 1: Introduction

My use of the Wisconsin law comes from Joel F. Handler and Ellen Jane Hollingsworth, *The Deserving Poor: A Study of Welfare Administration* (Chicago: Markham Publishing Co., 1971), and I rely on Katz,

Poverty and Policy in American History for a sense of how the poorhouse functioned.

Chapter 2: Inventing Social Security, 1935

The best sources on the origins of Social Security remain the reports of the Committee on Economic Security, including *Report to the President of the Committee on Economic Security* (Washington, D.C.: Government Printing Office, 1935) and *Social Security in America: The Factual Background of the Social Security Act as Summarized from Staff Reports to the Committee on Economic Security,* (Washington, D.C.: Government Printing Office, 1937). Also invaluable are the firsthand accounts and memoirs of the participants, including Edwin E. Witte, *The Development of the Social Security Act: A Memorandum on the History of the Committee on Economic Security and Drafting and Legislative History of the Social Security Act* (Madison: University of Wisconsin Press, 1963), Arthur J. Altmeyer, *The Formative Years of Social Security* (Madison: University of Wisconsin Press, 1966), Paul A. Raushenbush and Elizabeth Brandeis Raushenbush, "Our 'U.C.' Story" (Madison: privately printed, 1979), and J. Douglas Brown, *The Genesis of Social Security in America* (Princeton: Industrial Relations Section, 1969). The best contemporary appraisal of the Social Security Act is probably Paul H. Douglas, *Social Security in the United States: An Analysis and Appraisal of the Social Security Act* (New York: McGraw Hill, 1936). Irving Bernstein, *A Caring Society: The New Deal, the Worker, and the Great Depression* (Boston: Houghton Mifflin Co., 1985) does a nice job of recreating the Depression mood at the time of the Social Security Act's passage; so do William R. Brock, *Welfare, Democracy, and the New Deal* (New York: Cambridge University Press, 1988), and Jo Ann E. Argersinger, *Toward a New Deal in Baltimore: People and Government in the Great Depression* (Chapel Hill: The University of North Carolina Press, 1988).

The internecine battles over unemployment compensation can be traced through Paul Douglas's foreword to the Agathon Edition of Abraham Epstein, *Insecurity: A Challenge to America—A Study of Social Insurance in the United States and Abroad* (New York: Agathon Press, 1968), Daniel Nelson, *Unemployment Insurance: The American Experience, 1915–1935* (Madison: University of Wisconsin Press, 1969), and Part 3 of Edwin Witte, *Social Security Perspectives*, ed. Robert Lampman (Madison: University of Wisconsin Press, 1962).

Chapter 3: The Triumph of Social Security, 1936–1954

The genesis of the 1939 amendments can be found in Mark Leff, "Taxing the 'Forgotten Man': The Politics of Social Security Finance in the New Deal," *Journal of American History* 70 (September 1983): 359–81, Edward D. Berkowitz, "The First Social Security Crisis," *Prologue* 15 (Fall 1983): 133–49, and Brian Balogh, "Securing Support: The Emergence of the Social Security Board as a Political Actor, 1935–1939," in Critchlow and Hawley, eds., *Federal Social Policy: The Historical Dimension* (University Park: Pennsylvania State University Press, 1988). Leff has also written a definitive account of Social Security financing in the 1940s, "Speculating in Social Security Futures: The Perils of Payroll Tax Financing, 1939–1950," in Gerald D. Nash et al., eds., *Social Security: The First Half-Century* (Albuquerque: University of New Mexico Press, 1988). That same volume contains a perceptive essay by Blanche Coll on the fate of public assistance in these years, "Public Assistance: Reviving the Original Comprehensive Concept of Social Security," and a very interesting discussion of the circumstances surrounding the origins of Social Security by some pioneers who viewed the Social Security Act from the perspective of a half-century later. The Ohio episode can best be followed through Jill Quadagno and Madonna Harrington Meyer, "Organized Labor, State Structures, and Social Policy Development: A Case Study of Old-Age Assistance in Ohio, 1916–1940," *Social Problems* 36 (April 1989): 181–96. The Supreme Court opinion can be found in *Fiftieth Anniversary Edition, The Report of the Committee on Economic Security of 1935 and Other Basic Documents Relating to the Development of the Social Security Act* (Washington, D.C.: National Conference on Social Welfare, 1985.)

The best single source on Social Security developments in these years are the selections in William Haber and Wilbur J. Cohen, eds., *Readings in Social Security* (New York: Prentice-Hall, 1948), including Edwin E. Witte, "Development of Unemployment Compensation," reprinted from the *Yale Law Review*; Paul Raushenbush, "Federalization Threatens Experience Rating and State Laws," from an address to the American Photo-Engravers Association, October 1941; and the various reports of the 1948 advisory council, which are reprinted in full, such as Advisory Council on Social Security, *Old-Age and Survivors Insurance, Summary, Report to the Senate Committee on Finance*, 80th Cong., 2nd sess., (Washington, D.C.: Government Printing Office, 1948). A subsequent edition of the Haber and Cohen book of readings, published as *Social Security: Programs, Problems, and Pol-*

icies (Homewood, Ill.: Richard D. Irwin, 1960) is particularly good for the postwar consensus in Social Security.

A sense of the opposition to Social Security can be gleaned from Lewis Meriam, *Relief and Social Security* (Washington, D.C.: Brookings Institution, 1946).

On the Beveridge report and the English experience see William Beveridge, *Social Insurance and Allied Services* (New York: MacMillan Co., 1942) and José Harris, *William Beveridge: A Biography* (Oxford: Clarendon Press, 1977).

Chapter 4: The Day of Reckoning

A good account of the 1983 amendments is Paul Light, *Artful Work* (New York: Random House, 1985), which could be supplemented with Eric R. Kingson, "Financing Social Security: Agenda-Setting and the Enactment of the 1983 Amendments to the Social Security Act," *Policy Studies Journal* 13 (September 1984): 131–156. The flap over the Moynihan proposal can be studied through the newspaper clippings that are available through the National Academy of Social Insurance, Washington, D.C.

Chapter 5: Welfare's State, 1935–1967

Exploring this period of welfare's history, more than most topics in the area, requires that one consult primary sources. For the postwar emphasis on individual services see James Gilbert, *A Cycle of Outrage: America's Reaction to the Juvenile Delinquent in the 1950s* (New York: Oxford University Press, 1986). A valuable exploration of early developments in widows' pensions is Mark H. Leff, "Consensus for Reform: the Mothers' Pension Movement in the Progressive Era," *Social Service Review* 47 (September 1973): 397–415. An eloquent ode to the War on Poverty is Daniel Patrick Moynihan, *Maximum Feasible Misunderstanding* (New York: Free Press, 1969). Also instructive on the War on Poverty are Allen J. Matusow, *The Unraveling of America: A History of Liberalism in the 1960s* (New York: Harper and Row, 1984) and Peter Marris and Martin Rein, *Dilemmas of Social Reform: Poverty and Community Action in the United States* (Chicago: Aldine, 1973). My previous effort to understand such concepts as cultural deprivation is "The Politics of Mental Retardation in the Kennedy Administration," *Social Science Quarterly* 61 (June 1980): 128–142.

Chapter 6: Welfare Restated, 1967–1988

The work of the President's Commission on Income Maintenance is best understood through its report, *From Poverty amid Plenty: The American Paradox* (Washington, D.C.: Government Printing Office, 1969.) The Family Assistance Plan has generated a number of books, including Vincent J. Burke and Vee Burke, *Nixon's Good Deed: Welfare Reform* (New York: Columbia University Press, 1974), the best single-volume account, and Daniel Patrick Moynihan, *The Politics of a Guaranteed Annual Income: The Nixon Administration and the Family Assistance Plan* (New York: Vintage Books, 1973), which is immensely entertaining.

The welfare "mess" of the 1970s can be sympathetically understood by reading some of the overviews prepared by economists on the subject, including Henry Aaron, *On Social Welfare* (Cambridge, Mass.: Abt Books, 1980) and Lester M. Salamon, *Welfare: The Elusive Consensus* (New York: Praeger, 1978). A vivid account of the system from an administrator's point of view is Blanche Bernstein, *The Politics of Welfare: The New York City Experience* (Cambridge, Mass.: Abt Books, 1982). The role of the black family in this supposed mess remains a highly controversial matter, as is revealed in William Julius Wilson, *The Truly Disadvantaged: The Inner City, the Underclass, and Public Policy* (Chicago: University of Chicago Press, 1987). The best single-volume account of the effect of welfare on the family is the excellent and influential, David T. Ellwood, *Poor Support: Poverty in the American Family* (New York: Basic Books, 1988), which I have mined with considerable profit. My own thoughts on the Moynihan report and subsequent developments can be found in "Public History, Academic History, and Policy Analysis: A Case Study with Commentary," *The Public Historian* 4 (Fall 1988): 43–63. The report itself and a number of interesting commentaries are found in William L. Yancey and Lee Rainwater, *The Moynihan Report and the Politics of Controversy* (Boston: MIT Press, 1967).

The best introduction, by far, to the negative income tax experiments is Alicia H. Munnell, ed., *Lessons from the Income Maintenance Experiments, Proceedings of a Conference Held at Melvin Village, New Hampshire, September 1986*, published by the Federal Reserve Bank of Boston, conference series, No. 30 (1988?).

For the resurgence of conservative thought on welfare, the best source is Stuart Butler and Anna Kondratas, *Out of the Poverty Trap* (New York: Free Press, 1987), although the most famous source is Charles Murray, *Losing Ground* (New York: Basic Books, 1984). A very perceptive account of the difficulties in the negative income tax approach is Martin Anderson, *Welfare: The Political Economy of Welfare Reform in the United States* (Palo Alto, Calif.: Hoover Institution Press, 1978). See also Edward D. Berkowitz, "Changing the Meaning of Welfare Reform," in John Weicher, ed., *Maintaining the Safety Net: Income Redistribution Programs in the Reagan Administration* (Washington, D.C.: American Enterprise Institute, 1984), pp. 23–42.

The 1988 welfare amendments can be studied through several of the essays in Richard W. Couglin, ed., *Reforming Welfare: Lessons, Limits, and Choices* (Albuquerque: University of New Mexico Press, 1989), including Charles Lockhart, "The Contradictions in Public Assistance and the Prospect of Social Merging," John A. Daley, "Up from Dependency: The President's National Welfare Strategy," and A. Sidney Johnson III, "Welfare Reform: Prospects and Challenges." Also useful is Mark E. Rushefsky, *Public Policy in the United States: Toward the Twenty-first Century* (Pacific Grove, Calif.: Brooks/Cole Co., 1990), which uses the legislation as a case study of the policy process.

Chapter 7: Medicare and Health Policy, 1935–1989

Good discussions of Medicare can be found in Gaston V. Rimlinger, *Welfare Policy and Industrialization in Europe, America, and Russia* (New York: John Wiley and Sons, 1971), James L. Sundquist, *Politics and Policy: The Eisenhower, Kennedy, and Johnson Years* (Washington, D.C., The Brookings Institution, 1968), Rashi Fein, *The Search for a Health Insurance Policy* (Cambridge, Mass.: Harvard University Press, 1986), and Theodore Marmor, *The Politics of Medicare* (Chicago: Aldine Publishing Co., 1973).

As for the precursors to Medicare, I. S. Falk's original vision for health insurance can be discerned in Falk, *Security against Sickness* (Garden City, N.Y.: Doubleday, 1936). A spirited treatment of Blue Cross and its role in Medicare is Sylvia Law, *Blue Cross: What Went Wrong* (New Haven: Yale University Press, 1974). For other developments see Daniel S. Hirshfield, *The Lost Reform: The Campaign for Compulsory Health Insurance in the United States from 1932 to 1943* (Cambridge, Mass.: Harvard University Press, 1970). An illustration of the transformation of the hospital is David Rosner, *The Once Charitable Enterprise* (New York: Cambridge University Press, 1982).

A standard source on the development of medical research programs is Stephen P. Strickland, *Politics, Science, and Dread Disease: A Short History of United States Medical Research Policy* (Cambridge, Mass.: Harvard University Press, 1972), which might be supplemented with James T. Patterson, *The Dread Disease: Cancer and Modern American Culture* (Cambridge, Mass.: Harvard University Press, 1987).

For the particular case of mental health policy, see Gerald N. Grob, "The Forging of Mental Health Policy in America: World War II to New Frontier," *The Journal of the History of Medicine and Allied Sciences* 42 (October 1987): 410–446.

An accessible overview of health care costs is Carol M. McCarthy and Kenneth E. Thorpe, "Financing for Health Care," in Steven Jonas et al., eds., *Health Care Delivery in the United States*, 3rd ed. (Springfield, Ill.: Springer Publishing Co., 1986). Also valuable are the various articles in Carl J. Schramm, ed., *Health Care and Its Costs*, (New York: W. W. Norton and Co., 1987).

For the state experience with health care cost regulation see, The Maryland Health Services Cost Review Commission, "Hospital Rate Setting: Maryland's Experience, 1977–1983" (Baltimore, mimeo), and Kenneth E. Thorpe, "Does All-Payer Rate Setting Work? The Case of the New York Prospective Hospital Reimbursement Methodology," *Journal of Health Politics, Policy, and Law* 12 (Fall 1987): 391–408.

On prepaid group health see Lawrence D. Brown: *Politics and Health Care Organization: HMOs as Federal Policy* (Washington, D.C.: Brookings Institution, 1983), and Edward D. Berkowitz and Wendy Wolff, *Group Health Association: A Portrait of a Health Maintenance Organization* (Philadelphia: Temple University Press, 1988).

Chapter 8. Long-Term Care of the Welfare State

For contemporary perception of the long-term care issue see Tom Kenworthy, "House Girds for Fight on Medicare Expansion," *Washington Post*, June 6, 1988, p. 1: Molly Sinclair, "Coalition Backs Long-Term Care," *Washington Post*, October 6, 1987, p. A-10; and "Long-Term Care, An Idea That Can Elect the Next President. And Should," a pamphlet available through the Villers Foundation, Washington, D.C.; and Peter Osterlund, "Two Panels Probe Ways to Reshape Health-Care System," *Baltimore Sun*, September 11, 1989, p. A1.

Index

Index   211